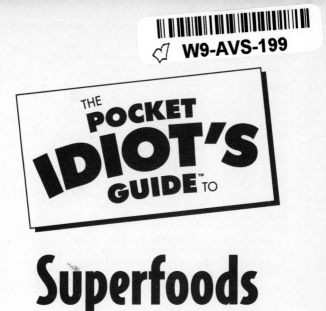

THE POCKET IDIOT'S GUIDE™ TO

Superfoods

by Heidi Reichenberger McIndoo,
M.S., R.D., L.D.N.

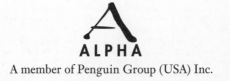

ALPHA

A member of Penguin Group (USA) Inc.

I dedicate this book to my beautiful little girl, Laila, in whom
I hope to instill a healthy enjoyment of a variety of foods.

ALPHA BOOKS

Published by the Penguin Group

Penguin Group (USA) Inc., 375 Hudson Street, New York, New York 10014, U.S.A.

Penguin Group (Canada), 10 Alcorn Avenue, Toronto, Ontario, Canada M4V 3B2 (a division of Pearson Penguin Canada Inc.)

Penguin Books Ltd, 80 Strand, London WC2R 0RL, England

Penguin Ireland, 25 St Stephen's Green, Dublin 2, Ireland (a division of Penguin Books Ltd)

Penguin Group (Australia), 250 Camberwell Road, Camberwell, Victoria 3124, Australia (a division of Pearson Australia Group Pty Ltd)

Penguin Books India Pvt Ltd, 11 Community Centre, Panchsheel Park, New Delhi—110 017, India

Penguin Group (NZ), cnr Airborne and Rosedale Roads, Albany, Auckland 1310, New Zealand (a division of Pearson New Zealand Ltd)

Penguin Books (South Africa) (Pty) Ltd, 24 Sturdee Avenue, Rosebank, Johannesburg 2196, South Africa

Penguin Books Ltd, Registered Offices: 80 Strand, London WC2R 0RL, England

International Standard Book Number: 978-1-59257-612-8
Library of Congress Catalog Card Number: 2006934453

09 08 07   8 7 6 5 4 3 2 1

Interpretation of the printing code: The rightmost number of the first series of numbers is the year of the book's printing; the rightmost number of the second series of numbers is the number of the book's printing. For example, a printing code of 07-1 shows that the first printing occurred in 2007.

Printed in the United States of America

Note: This publication contains the opinions and ideas of its author. It is intended to provide helpful and informative material on the subject matter covered. It is sold with the understanding that the author and publisher are not engaged in rendering professional services in the book. If the reader requires personal assistance or advice, a competent professional should be consulted.

The author and publisher specifically disclaim any responsibility for any liability, loss, or risk, personal or otherwise, which is incurred as a consequence, directly or indirectly, of the use and application of any of the contents of this book.

Most Alpha books are available at special quantity discounts for bulk purchases for sales promotions, premiums, fund-raising, or educational use. Special books, or book excerpts, can also be created to fit specific needs.

For details, write: Special Markets, Alpha Books, 375 Hudson Street, New York, NY 10014.

Contents

1 Superfoods: More Powerful Than
   a Locomotive   1

2 Bountiful Berries   11

3 Eat a Rainbow: Super Vegetables   31

4 Drink to Your Health   63

5 Soy and Yogurt   81

6 Protein Power   105

7 Fields of Dreams   123

8 Sometimes You Feel Like a Nut   137

9 The Spices of Life   153

10 How Sweet It Is   165

Appendixes

A Glossary   175

B Dietary Reference Intakes for
   Selected Vitamins and Minerals   187

C Internet Resources   195

D Recommended Books   199

   Index   203

Introduction

With all the advances in modern science, you'd think we'd be so much healthier than we were 20, 30, or even 50 years ago. While we certainly are living longer, and many fatal diseases are all but distant memories, in a way we're sicker than ever. Chronic diseases like cardiovascular disease and diabetes are rising at alarming rates. And even more frightening is that many of these diseases are being diagnosed at younger and younger ages. Type 2 diabetes historically developed around midlife, in a person's 40s or 50s, but now men and women in their 20s are being diagnosed. In addition, teens are increasingly being diagnosed with pre-diabetes. And it's not because of improvements in diagnosing.

I believe part of the reason for the increased prevalence of these debilitating and sometimes life-threatening illnesses is that Americans have gotten away from whole foods; there's a tremendous reliance on processed and convenience foods. I see this every day when I counsel patients. When asked how often they eat fast food or convenience foods, they answer me in "times per day." However, when I ask how often fruits or vegetables are part of their diet, the answer is usually in terms of "times per week or month." How sad.

Whole foods like whole grains, fruits, vegetables, and more are created in nature with a certain nutritional profile. What I mean is that each food has its own unique combination of nutrients. While every nutrient provides its own health benefit, when nutrients are eaten together, the benefits far outweigh what each could do on its own. Whole foods usually contain several nutrients that work together in this way. For example, peanuts contain healthy fats as well as vitamin E, a fat-soluble vitamin that needs fat to be absorbed and used properly. Alternatively, in the processing of convenience and fast foods, many nutrients are removed or lost, and we lose that synergistic activity between the naturally occurring nutrients.

In an ideal world, we would all go back to whole foods and steer clear of processed foods. But for many reasons, time constraints being a significant one, that's probably not going to happen. So the next-best thing would be achieving a healthy balance between the two—for example, a diet filled with nutrient-packed whole foods that's peppered here and there with slightly processed convenience foods.

And this is where superfoods come in. I'll be the first to tell you that all foods can fit into a healthy diet. But in a part-processed, part-whole foods menu, superfoods are a great fit. Like all whole foods, superfoods contain a substantial amount of beneficial components. But superfoods really stand out because on top of that, the nutrients they do contain are really designed to get the most out of that synergistic action.

If you'd like to start eating healthier but can't or don't want to do a sudden 180° in your eating, adding superfoods to your usual diet is a great first step. They will certainly give you the most bang for your buck.

Maybe you already eat fairly healthfully and are just looking for that little something more. A superfood here and there can definitely help put you over the top, nutritionally speaking.

Or it could be that you already eat all of these wonderful foods and want to learn just how good they are for you.

Whatever your reason, the bottom line is that this book is filled with nutritious and delicious foods that nourish your body and satisfy your appetite.

Super Sidebars

Scattered throughout this book are boxes or sidebars that offer extra information to provide you with a better understanding of an idea or warn you about something requiring extra caution.

def•i•ni•tion

When it comes to nutrition, scientists like to use all kinds of big words. And sometimes there are words you hear all the time but just were never quite sure exactly what they meant. These boxes will help translate all the fancy mumbo-jumbo into everyday terms.

Kryptonite

These boxes offer a warning of some kind. It may be as simple as a suggestion to help you control your calories, or it could be advice to avoid certain foods altogether. You never know, so it's a good idea to check them out.

Super Knowledge

These boxes give you extra details about foods mentioned in the chapter. They may include tips on how to store the foods or provide extra nutritional material.

Acknowledgments

As a food lover and registered dietitian, this book was a perfect fit for me. I'd like to thank my literary agent, Marilyn Allen, who felt the same way and helped me in the process of getting started. Thank you to Tom Stevens, my editor, who was always there with an answer to my many questions.

Special thanks to my mom, Sandy Swadley, for being my first reviewer and editor. Thank you to my baby girl, Laila, for amusing herself (and me) while Mommy worked, and for all the hugs, grins, and giggles when I needed them. And certainly thank you to my husband, Sean, for his help and support and for reminding me to, or—to be more accurate—making me take breaks and relax.

Special Thanks to the Technical Reviewer

The Pocket Idiot's Guide™ to Superfoods was reviewed by an expert who double-checked the accuracy of what you'll learn here, to help us ensure that this book gives you everything you need to know about the benefits of superfoods. Special thanks are extended to Peggy O'Shea Kochenbach, M.B.A., R.D., L.D.N.

Peggy O'Shea Kochenbach, M.B.A., R.D., L.D.N., has over 10 years of experience providing communications expertise and is currently a vice president with Cone, Inc., in Boston. There, she has developed nutrition-related programming and has assisted in communicating health and nutrition messages for companies in the food and nutrition, nonprofit, and health-care sectors. Her past experience includes both group teaching and private counseling in the areas of weight management, corporate wellness, cardiac rehabilitation, and clinical dietetics, including work as chief clinical dietitian at a Boston-area hospital. In 2005, she was awarded the Recognized Young Dietitian of the Year award and is currently the president of the Massachusetts Dietetic Association.

Trademarks

All terms mentioned in this book that are known to be or are suspected of being trademarks or service marks have been appropriately capitalized. Alpha Books and Penguin Group (USA) Inc. cannot attest to the accuracy of this information. Use of a term in this book should not be regarded as affecting the validity of any trademark or service mark.

Superfoods: More Powerful Than a Locomotive

In This Chapter

- Superwhats?
- The good, the bad, and the not-so-ugly
- Don't deny yourself
- Variety, variety, variety

Superfoods, functional foods, power foods. Whatever name you prefer, they're all pretty much the same thing. Superfoods are foods that go above and beyond the basic nutrition of vitamins and minerals. So, before we get into the specifics of all the tremendous benefits these foods have to offer, first a bit on how they fit into our diet.

"Good" and "Bad" Foods

It's common to hear, when people discuss food, the terms "good" and "bad" in reference to specific foods. As a registered dietitian and food lover, that really bothers me. If someone is talking about how a food tastes, that's fine—there are certainly plenty of bad-tasting foods out there (along with all the great-tasting ones), and if someone wants to warn me against eating something with a less-than-appealing taste, please do. What bothers me is when these descriptions are used to suggest whether we should eat a food or not—along the lines of "It's bad for me, so I won't eat it" or "I don't like it, but I'll eat it because it's good for me." In that sense, I don't believe there are good and bad foods. There are simply foods we should eat more frequently and those we should eat less frequently.

Why do I feel that way, you might ask? For a number of reasons. And in no particular order, I'm going to share them with you. First, the food lover in me has a hard time with the idea of completely denying yourself the foods you like simply because they are less than healthy. While eating is indispensable for maintaining life, food serves many more purposes than simply acting as the fuel that makes the engine of our body run. Food should be savored and enjoyed. And doing that requires eating foods you like. However, fully realizing the potential of this way of thinking requires a bit of adventurousness and a willingness to try new foods.

Another pet peeve of mine is when someone tells me they dislike fruits and vegetables, for example, and then admits, after I offer a long list of them, that they've never tried most of them. In order to fit the foods that may not offer much nutritionally into your diet, you still need to eat a good amount of healthy foods. And allowing for maximum enjoyment of these foods may mean continually trying new foods and different ways to prepare foods to find what you like best.

When we designate certain foods as "bad," we often try to eliminate them from our diet. But complete denial, or at least attempted denial, of our favorite foods is never a good idea. It leads to feeling deprived. In addition to taking the fun out of eating, feelings of deprivation often lead to binges. Bingeing can cause guilt because you ate something you feel you shouldn't have and most likely ate too much of it. Now you're stuck in an unending cycle of abstinence and gluttony, neither of which is conducive to healthy eating. A much healthier way to go about it is to find ways to occasionally fit in the less-than-healthy foods. Allowing yourself to go out for an ice cream cone every couple weeks is certainly more enjoyable and better for you than inhaling a pint or two of ice cream. This leads to feeling guilty, and then restricting yourself until you can't take it anymore and you find yourself back at the freezer digging around for more super-premium double-chocolate-chip ice cream.

And finally, many of the foods people describe as bad often have a redeeming quality. For example, the ice cream above can be a good source of calcium. There are plenty of other foods that provide as much or more calcium along with a lot fewer calories, fat, and sugar. For this reason there's no official recommendation for a daily amount of ice cream a person needs, because technically you don't "need" any. But an occasional indulgence from the food group I refer to as "Others," which includes pies, chips, etc., can fit into an eating plan filled primarily with healthy foods.

A Healthy Eating Plan

What makes up a healthy eating plan, you ask? Choosing foods from all five food groups: grains, vegetables, fruits, milk, and meat and beans form the basis for a nutritious diet. The USDA developed My Pyramid to explain the different food groups and how many servings from each group you need, based on your gender, age, and activity level. The recommendations for how much to choose from each food group are also based on the nutrient content of the food. For example, dairy foods such as low-fat milk, yogurt, and cheese are excellent sources of calcium. Therefore, one factor considered in the recommendation of three cups a day is the amount of calcium in one cup in comparison to how much your body needs.

Here's a sample of the My Pyramid recommendations for an adult eating 2,000 calories per day. To find out your specific needs, go to www. mypyramid.gov and plug in your age, gender, and activity amount. You'll get specific suggestions for how many servings of each food group you should be eating each day, as well as tips and information about each food group.

Food Group	Number of Servings per Day	Serving Size
Grains	6 ounces; at least 3 should be whole-grain	1 ounce is about 1 slice of bread; 1 cup of cold cereal; or 1/2 cup of cooked pasta, rice, or cereal
Vegetables	2½ cups	1 cup of raw or cooked veggies, 1 cup of juice, or 2 cups of leafy greens
Fruits	2 cups	1 cup of fruit or 100% fruit juice or 1/2 cup of dried fruit
Milk	3 cups	1 cup of milk or yogurt, 1½ ounces of natural cheese, or 2 ounces of processed cheese
Meat and Beans	5½ ounces	1 ounce of meat, poultry, or fish; 1/4 cup of cooked dry beans; 1 egg; 1 tablespoon of peanut butter; or 1/2 ounce of nuts

Each of the five food groups has its own unique benefits, and eating more from one group doesn't make up for skipping another group. A healthy diet includes foods from the grain group for getting fiber and many B vitamins; the vegetable group for getting vitamins A and K; the fruit group for getting fiber and vitamin C; the milk group for getting calcium, protein, and vitamin D; and the meat and bean group for getting protein, iron, and zinc. These are just a few examples and by no means a complete list of all the nutrients each food group contains. Eliminating one group from your diet not only removes all the delicious foods in that group, but it also robs your body of all of the important nutrients those foods contain.

Often foods aren't so straightforward as to which group they belong in. Therefore, it's tough to know what a serving is. Fortunately, all packaged foods you buy have nutrition facts labels. These tell you what one serving is and so much more. You can learn information such as how many calories or how much fat one serving contains, as well as the content of several other nutrients including fiber, sugar, and sodium. Plus, if applicable, the nutrition facts label will tell you what *Percent Daily Value* of certain vitamins one serving of the food provides. The nutrition facts labels can be very helpful when trying to make healthy food choices.

This brings me back to the idea of trying new foods. If you think you're missing out on a food group because you don't like the foods it contains, get daring—find some foods in that group you've never tasted and give them a try. Or get creative in the kitchen and try new ways to prepare foods that in the past haven't wowed you. That's step one on your trip to a healthier you. And just wait until you learn about step two—it's "super"!

def•i•ni•tion

> **Percent Daily Value** is the amount of the recommended needs of the nutrient that the named food provides. It is based on the needs of a person eating 2,000 calories per day.

The Importance of Variety

Superfoods come from all the food groups, and they definitely fall into the category of foods to eat more of because they contain compounds that, while not necessary for the everyday workings of your body, can improve your health. These compounds can actually help prevent an assortment of diseases, too.

To decrease your risk of cancer, heart disease, *diabetes*, Alzheimer's, and more, wouldn't you do all you could? And what if part of doing so meant enjoying delicious foods and drinks every day? Including a variety of superfoods in your diet on a regular basis lets you do just that.

def•i•ni•tion

Diabetes is a chronic disease characterized by high levels of glucose, or sugar, in the blood. Consistent blood sugar elevation can damage your kidneys and eyes and cause other complications.

I know what you're thinking, but before you go and start trying to make a daily menu from the 25 foods I discuss in this book or concoct some crazy recipe with strawberries, carrots, tofu, and grape juice, just wait. These are not magic bullets that must be consumed every day or to the exclusion of other foods. The foods I discuss are healthful when included as part of a balanced diet that includes an assortment of foods.

Kryptonite

If a little is good, a lot isn't necessarily better. Most of us have heard that boring term—moderate portions—when it comes to dieting and losing weight. Believe it or not, that expression can be applied to healthy food as well. While a moderate portion of cranberries or soymilk might be a bit larger than a moderate portion of, say, french fries, the phrase still holds true. Overdosing on some healthy foods could lead to weight gain, while too much of others may have more serious consequences I'll describe in detail within the following pages.

You may have picked up this book for any number of reasons, but a common thread throughout them all is an interest in your health. So always keep in mind that the key to healthy eating is choosing a variety of foods from all of the food groups each day.

The Least You Need to Know

- While they may not help us leap tall buildings, superfoods do offer us many super powers.
- Stop thinking of foods as good and bad (unless it's how they taste, of course).
- Foods can help prevent disease.
- A moderate amount of a variety of foods from all food groups is the key to a healthy diet.

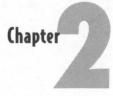

Chapter 2

Bountiful Berries

In This Chapter

- Phytochemicals aren't for sprinkling on your lawn
- Enjoy fruit year-round every day
- Those pretty colors do more than just give you something to look at
- Flavonoids aren't a video game from the '80s

No matter if they are big or small, tart or sweet, summer's juicy berries are full of fabulous flavors and bright colors. And it's those colors, those blues and reds, that give berries many of their healthful properties. Strawberries, blueberries, cranberries, and cherries contain special nutrients called phytochemicals.

Phytochemicals are compounds found in plants that aren't essential for the body to function but are beneficial in improving health or decreasing the risk of certain diseases. Berries are packed with phytochemicals, fiber, and an assortment of vitamins and minerals to help cure what ails us or to prevent the ailing in the first place.

The different berries share many of the nutrients found within them, meaning you can obtain most of the health benefits I'm telling you about by including any one of them in your diet. However, they each also have properties unique to themselves. Ideally you should try to eat a variety of all of them on a regular basis.

One group of phytochemicals found in berries is *antioxidants*. While we're born with natural defenses against *oxidative stress*, as we age our defenses weaken and the stress increases, making it doubly important to obtain adequate antioxidants from our diets.

def•i•ni•tion

> **Antioxidants** protect our bodies' cells from the oxidative stress and damage done by substances known as free radicals. They may possibly reduce the risks of certain cancers and age-related diseases.
>
> **Oxidative stress** is the damage done to our bodies' tissue and cells by free radicals. The process is not unlike the way rust forms in the dings and dents on our cars.

For most of the country, summer is the peak season for getting plump, flavorful, fresh berries. But fortunately for all of us, we can get frozen berries, and some canned, year-round. And don't think you're settling for less than the best by getting some icy fruit from the frozen-foods department. Frozen fruit is just as nutritious and sometimes more so than fresh. That's because in most cases the berries are flash frozen as soon as they're picked and kept frozen until you thaw them, preserving all the nutrients and flavor. That goes for canned fruit as well. Fruit canners process and can their berries as soon after picking as possible. Compare that to fresh produce, which gets packaged up, loaded onto a truck, delivered to your local store or farmers market, bought by you, and then finally brought to your house to enjoy. The freshness and quality of your fresh fruit depends on how long each of those steps takes.

Kryptonite

When buying canned fruit, choose fruit canned in water or juice versus syrup. This will save you unnecessary sugar and calories. If you can't find it canned in water or juice, simply rinse off the sugary syrup before digging in.

As a whole, berries are very low in calories, containing just 50–75 calories in a half cup. They are virtually fat- and sodium-free. Those factors alone should be enough to convince you to start eating them. Whether you're watching your salt intake, your fat intake, or your waistline, berries are a great choice to include in your diet. Add in the fact that they are absolutely delicious and I think we've got a sale!

The Blueberry

Remember Violet Beauregarde blowing up into a giant blueberry in the book and movie *Charlie and the Chocolate Factory?* Well, thank goodness that can't happen in real life or we'd be in trouble. Blueberries are full of good, not harm.

Nutrition Information for ½ Cup of Blueberries

Calories	40
Total Fat	0 grams
Saturated Fat	0 grams
Trans Fat	0 grams
Cholesterol	0 milligrams
Sodium	0 milligrams
Total Carbohydrate	11 grams
Dietary Fiber	1 gram
Sugars	7 grams
Protein	1 gram
Vitamin C	10% Daily Value
Iron	2% Daily Value

First, let's get something straight. I'm not talking about those dried-up little specks of blue matter you find in a muffin mix or your breakfast cereal. I mean real, whole blueberries. And, like I said before, it doesn't matter if they are fresh, frozen, or canned—as long as you include them on your grocery list. Neither a tight budget nor the time of year is an excuse to not have blueberries.

Blueberries really are a superstar when it comes to antioxidants, particularly wild blueberries. In fact, a test called Oxygen Radical Absorbance Capacity (OREC) showed that 100 grams or just over three quarters of a cup of wild blueberries contain 2,400 ORAC units. That's more antioxidant activity than was found in a serving of more than 20 other fresh fruits tested.

Super Knowledge

While it's not an official recommendation, scientists estimate a daily intake of 3,000 to 5,000 ORAC units should be adequate to prevent or slow some age-related changes that cause mental and physical decline. Scientists estimate that the average person consumes around 1,200 ORAC units daily.

Responsible for all of this power are a few specific components called *flavonoids*. There are more than 4,000 subcategories of flavonoids based on structure.

These categories include flavonols, anthocyanidins (which have been shown to improve the health of blood vessels), and proanthocyanidins (which may have a role in decreasing your risk of cardiovascular disease and cancer, and may also help protect against urinary tract infections). The flavonol found in blueberries is *myricetin*.

def•i•ni•tion

Flavonoids are the most powerful and abundant phytochemical group in your diet.

Myricetin is a flavonoid shown in studies to have anti-inflammatory and anti-cancer properties. It's found in vegetables and fruits (primarily berries), grapes, parsley, and spinach.

Now you know what's doing all the work in those tiny little spheres, but exactly what kind of work are they doing for you? Like I said, blueberries are tremendously powerful and offer many benefits to your health. Including blueberries as a frequent part of your diet may improve motor skills and even reverse the short-term memory loss associated with aging and age-related diseases like Alzheimer's. These improvements were seen with eating the equivalent of one cup of blueberries per day. It's suspected that the anthocyanidins are the responsible party in this case. Anthocyanidins also give blueberries their beautiful deep-blue hue.

If you've ever suffered through the discomfort and annoyance of a urinary tract infection (UTI), keep reading. These infections are caused by bacteria clinging to the inner walls of the urinary tract and then multiplying. The proanthocyanidins in blueberries prevent the bacteria from sticking. If the bacteria can't attach somewhere, it can't multiply. While it's too soon to say for sure that blueberries will prevent UTIs, this finding is the big first step in that direction.

While more studies must be done to show direct evidence, some links between blueberry intake and cancer prevention have been seen. Wild blueberries may be beneficial in preventing or slowing the early stages of cancer development. And in lab studies, blueberry juice was shown to greatly slow the growth of breast and cervical cancer.

The Strawberry

There aren't too many desserts you can include in a list of healthful foods. But strawberry shortcake might just fit the bill. Sure, there's the whole cake thing, but a simple biscuit or some angel food cake isn't that bad. Then there's the cream, but a little dab once in a while won't hurt you. Finally, the piece de resistance, those fabulous strawberries.

Nutrition Information for ½ Cup of Strawberries

Calories	25
Total Fat	0 grams
Saturated Fat	0 grams
Trans Fat	0 grams
Cholesterol	0 milligrams
Sodium	0 milligrams

continues

Nutrition Information for ¹/₂ Cup of Strawberries (continued)

Total Carbohydrate	6 grams
Dietary Fiber	2 grams
Sugars	4 grams
Protein	1 gram
Vitamin C	80% Daily Value
Calcium	2% Daily Value
Iron	2% Daily Value

Like their summertime buddy the blueberry, strawberries are filled to the brim with antioxidant power. Specifically, the flavonoids found in strawberries are proanthocyanidins, anthocyanidins, and *quercetin*. They also contain the phytochemical *ellagic acid*.

def•i•ni•tion

Quercetin is considered the major flavonoid in a diet. Those who eat the most foods containing it have a decreased risk of asthma and lung cancer, and lower death from heart disease.

Ellagic acid is a polyphenol that has antioxidant properties and helps reduce the risk of certain cancers.

In addition to all of these fancy words, strawberries contain another powerful antioxidant, vitamin C. That's right, good old vitamin C is an antioxidant. One cup of strawberries or about eight medium berries contains 84 milligrams of vitamin C. That's more of the disease-fighting vitamin than a whole orange has. We may feel it helps us get better when we're sick, but it does so much more.

And remember our old buddy ORAC from earlier? Eight medium strawberries contain 1,540 ORAC units. Not quite as much as the blueberries, but still enough to get you well on your way to 3,000–5,000 units a day.

When it comes to the health of your heart, consider tossing some juicy strawberries into your menu regularly. In addition to vitamin C, strawberries contain the vitamin *folate*, the mineral *potassium*, and fiber. All four of these nutrients help protect your heart and cardiovascular system from disease.

def•i•ni•tion

Folate is a B-vitamin that plays a big role in preventing birth defects and producing red blood cells. It is also called folic acid.

Potassium is a mineral involved in controlling blood pressure and regulating muscle contractions.

Homocysteine is an amino acid found in your blood. High levels of it coincide with a higher risk of heart disease.

People who regularly eat strawberries tend to have lower levels of *homocysteine* as well as lower blood pressure than those who don't eat strawberries. Low measures of both of these are two signs of good heart health.

Folate performs many functions in your body. One is lowering homocysteine levels in your blood. Just eight medium strawberries provide almost 20 percent of your needed folate.

In addition to possibly helping fend off the common cold, vitamin C is a powerful antioxidant that's been shown to have a link with decreased rates of death from heart disease. Adequate vitamin C in your diet may also help lower your blood levels of C-reactive protein. This is another marker for heart disease.

Strawberries are also a good source of fiber. We've probably all been told to get more fiber into our diets. But why? Why not is a better question. Fiber helps to fill us up so we feel satisfied after eating. But that's really a minor bonus compared to all its other benefits. In terms of heart disease alone, folks who eat higher amounts of fiber have lower risks of both heart disease and high blood pressure. Lowering your blood pressure is a double-whammy when it comes to your health. High blood pressure, or hypertension as it's also known, is a disease all on its own. Therefore, lowering it is an improvement in your health. But high blood pressure is also a risk factor for heart disease, so lower blood pressure means a lower risk of heart disease.

The fiber in strawberries is the soluble kind, which means it helps to lower your cholesterol—yet another way strawberry fiber boosts your heart health. Eight medium strawberries provide 3 grams of fiber. It may not seem like a lot, but it adds up over the course of a day filled with a variety of healthy food choices like fruits, veggies, and whole grains.

Super Knowledge

About 25 to 35 grams of fiber per day is what the National Research Council recommends. These are the same folks who determine the RDAs and DRIs.

Potassium content is another way strawberries work to get that blood pressure down. One of potassium's jobs in your body is to regulate blood pressure. Eating a selection of foods high in potassium and low in sodium can help reduce your risk of high blood pressure and, in doing so, reduce your risk of having a stroke. In fact, there's an entire diet built around that concept called the DASH (Dietary Approaches to Stop Hypertention) diet.

And finally, those awesome antioxidants are at it again. Quercetin and anthocyanins help to slow blood clotting. Clots in blood vessels are the cause of strokes and heart attacks. By decreasing the clotting, you're lowering the risk of these scary, debilitating, and often-deadly events. Plus antioxidants help to keep your blood vessels flexible, yet another way of lowering your risk for heart disease.

In addition to the many ways strawberries are good for your heart, these rosy little berries are being investigated for their role against cancer. We already know strawberries are an excellent source of vitamin C. And while it's too soon to say flat out that strawberries decrease your risk of cancer, it is known that vitamin C has been linked with lower rates of stomach, cervical, and breast cancers. So it's likely that eating strawberries regularly can produce similar benefits.

And remember that term "ellagic acid" several paragraphs ago? I didn't forget about it. Its involvement in your health has to do with cancer prevention. This is another one of those "still early in the research" kind of things. But in lab studies, ellagic acid shows promise in slowing both the development and growth of cancer cells.

Certainly there's still much more work to be done. But it's clear that strawberries and good health go hand in hand.

The Cranberry

The most well-known benefit of cranberries is with regard to urinary tract infections. But before I get to that, I want to go over some of the lesser-known works of that little berry many of us see only alongside a turkey in November.

Nutrition Information for ½ Cup of Cranberries

Calories	30
Total Fat	0 grams
Saturated Fat	0 grams
Trans Fat	0 grams
Cholesterol	0 milligrams
Sodium	0 milligrams
Total Carbohydrate	7 grams
Dietary Fiber	2 grams
Sugars	5 grams
Protein	0 grams
Vitamin C	10% Daily Value

Super Knowledge

Americans eat around 400 million pounds of cranberries each year. Twenty percent or about 80 million pounds of those are eaten the week of Thanksgiving.

Just like the other berries, cranberries are filled with a variety of flavonoids that do remarkable work toward improving your health. The antioxidants in these deep-red berries may protect your heart by raising your *HDL* cholesterol. In addition, cranberries have been shown to slow the *oxidation* of *LDL* cholesterol.

def•i•ni•tion

HDL stands for high-density-lipoprotein. Referred to as "good" cholesterol, HDL helps rid cholesterol from your body.

LDL stands for low-density-lipoprotein. Often called "bad" cholesterol, it's responsible for the plaque buildup that narrows your arteries and could lead to a heart attack or stroke.

Oxidation is a chemical reaction in your body that produces free radicals and damages your cells.

More science showing good reasons to include cranberries in your diet is still underway. Early reports show promise that cranberries may be a powerful weapon against cancer. In addition, cranberries could protect the brain from the damaging effects of aging. They do have quite a high ORAC value. Just 3½ ounces of fresh berries contains 1,750 ORAC units.

Now, for what we've all been waiting for, preventing the dreaded urinary tract infection. The proanthocyanidins in cranberries, similar to their blueberry cousins, prevent the bacteria that cause urinary tract infections from sticking to the urinary tract wall. If the bacteria can't stick, it can't grow. If it can't grow, it can't make us sick. It appears that an 8-ounce glass of cranberry juice cocktail twice a day is all we need for this.

Kryptonite

While a little juice may be a good thing, more isn't necessarily better. Juices contain many nutritive properties, but they also contain a fair amount of sugar. Drinking more than one or two glasses per day raises your sugar and therefore calorie intake and could lead to unwanted weight gain.

Those scientists are smart folks. They thought that if cranberries could keep bacteria from sticking to the urinary tract wall, maybe it could stop it from sticking elsewhere. Well, sure enough, it seems that cranberry juice inhibits bacteria from sticking to your teeth. This bacteria leads to cavities and gum disease. So some cranberry juice every day may help to keep the dentist away (and his awful drill, too).

It used to be thought that stomach ulcers were caused by stress and stomach acid. Increasingly, it appears that these ulcers develop from bacteria called H. pylori sticking to the stomach wall. I'm sure you can figure out where I'm going with this one. Cranberries may be helpful in decreasing the chances that H. pylori will stick to the stomach wall, therefore lowering the likelihood of ulcer development. And if that's not good enough for you, the ulcer-causing H. pylori has been linked to gastritis, reflux disease, and stomach cancer. So even if you've never had an ulcer, preventing H. pylori from doing its thing can benefit you in a number of ways.

The Cherry

When it comes to cherries, we've got two basic types to talk about. Sweet cherries are the ones you find in the produce section of the market in June. Sour or tart cherries aren't usually available fresh because they are too sour to eat that way. You can find them frozen, canned, or dried, and they're most often used for baking. Sour cherry juice is also available.

Nutrition Information for ½ Cup of Cherries

Calories	45
Total Fat	0 grams
Saturated Fat	0 grams
Trans Fat	0 grams
Cholesterol	0 milligrams
Sodium	0 milligrams
Total Carbohydrate	12 grams
Dietary Fiber	2 grams
Sugars	9 grams
Protein	1 gram
Vitamin C	8% Daily Value
Iron	2% Daily Value

Like the berries, cherries contain a whole host of phytochemicals and antioxidants. They also have been measured for their ORAC capacity. Three

and a half ounces of sweet cherries contain 580
ORAC units. However, the same amount of dried
tart cherries contains a whopping 6,800 ORAC
units. Now if you remember back a few pages, I
said blueberries had more antioxidant power than
other fruits, and that's still true when it comes to
fresh fruit—but dried fruits are a different category.
What does that mean for you? It means go ahead
and enjoy a variety of fresh and dried fruits to maximize your food power.

Because cherries contain many of the same phytochemicals as berries, many of the health benefits
are similar. Bing cherries, the ones usually found
fresh, may help decrease your risk of heart disease
in a number of ways. Eating them on a regular
basis has been shown to lower blood levels of three
different heart disease markers. One of these is
C-reactive protein, a blood protein that rises with
inflammation associated with heart disease, arthritis, and cancer. In addition, elevated levels of
C-reactive protein are a warning sign of a stroke,
as well as other cardiovascular ailments.

Arthritis and gout are two common problems
involving tissue inflammation. Just 20 cherries
contain 25 milligrams of anthocyanidins. That's
enough to stop the enzymes that cause your tissue
from becoming inflamed and therefore prevent the
pain from occurring.

Having trouble sleeping? Try trading in your
warm milk for a handful of cherries. Sour cherries
contain large amounts of melatonin. You may have
heard of this one. Melatonin is a hormone involved

in the regulation of sleep-and-wake cycles. That means it can help improve natural sleep patterns. The cherry is one of the few foods that contain melatonin in a form that the body can easily use, and it contains much more than any other food in which it's been measured. Melatonin also has anti-oxidant capabilities, which means it can help fight the damage *free radicals* do to your brain, cardio-vascular system, and immune system. Therefore it can help slow some of the signs of aging. As we age, our bodies produce fewer antioxidants on their own but more free radicals. So consuming adequate anti-oxidants in your diet is crucial, especially as you grow older.

Here's another bonus not addressed with any of the berries: possible diabetes control. Cherries contain a couple of specific anthocyanins with big, long scientific names you don't want to know. These components have been shown to stimulate *insulin* secretion.

def•i•ni•tion

> **Free radicals** are the result of the normal chemical reactions in the body. They damage your cells and accelerate the development of age-related and other diseases.
>
> **Insulin** is the hormone responsible for lowering your blood sugar by transporting the sugar from your blood to the various body tissues that need it for fuel.

By stimulating insulin secretion, these components can help to lower blood sugar levels in those with diabetes. If you happen to have this condition, I'm not telling you to skip your medicine and just eat some cherries. More research needs to be done, and until then you should continue the treatment plan you and your doctor have developed. However, cherries could certainly fit into a well-balanced diabetic eating pattern.

The Least You Need to Know

- Blueberries have more antioxidant power than 20 other tested fruits.
- All fruit is healthy, whether fresh, frozen, or canned.
- Don't save cranberries just for Thanksgiving—enjoy their benefits year-round.
- Cherries may help with insomnia problems.

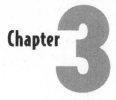

Eat a Rainbow: Super Vegetables

In This Chapter

- Extremely low-calorie content and high-phytochemical content makes vegetables the most nutrient-dense food group
- Cooked tomato products like ketchup and tomato sauce on pizza are good for us …
- Pumpkins and sweet potatoes are for more than just sitting next to a roasted turkey in November
- Can we cure the common cold?

Just like berries and all other fruits, vegetables are loaded with antioxidants. The antioxidants in veggies may take the form of vitamins, minerals, phytochemicals (such as flavonoids and *carotenoids*), and more.

def•i•ni•tion

Carotenoids are strong antioxidants that may lower the risk of heart disease, some types of cancer, age-related eye diseases, and lung diseases. They are responsible for the vibrant orange and red colors of many vegetables.

In general, vegetables, especially the brightly or deeply colored ones, protect our bodies from the same stresses and damage from which berries protect us. The more intense the color, the better. So deep-green broccoli provides more health benefits than does light celery. Bright orange carrots are more powerful than pale yellow corn. I'm not saying that celery and corn are unhealthy, not at all. All fruits and vegetables are nutritious. Some are just more so than others.

You thought berries were low in calories? Well, wait until you read this! Most veggies have between 15 and 25 calories per half cup. Spinach is one exception. A half cup of raw spinach has only 3 calories. That's right, I said 3. And they are loaded with fiber but contain little to no fat or sodium. For this reason, veggies are great to eat when trying to drop a few pounds. The fiber helps fill you up, among other bonuses, but without the calories other foods offer. For example, for the same calories as 1 cup of white rice, you'd need to eat 8½ cups of cauliflower! In fact, I often tell weight-loss clients while controlling portions of other foods to go ahead and eat unlimited amounts of veggies. Chances are you'll fill up long before you could eat enough to gain or maintain weight.

Now, before I get into the fun stuff, I want to make one thing clear. All these wonderful colors and foods I'm talking about are those occurring in nature. So when I'm going on about how great red foods such as peppers and tomatoes are, it's no mistake that I don't mention those sugary fruit-punch drinks. And gummi bears haven't been accidentally left out of this list. I'm not saying these foods shouldn't be eaten; I'm just saying that if it doesn't grow from a tree or out of the ground, it most likely won't give you the benefits I'm talking about on the following pages.

Radical Reds

I'll bet you could think of a list of foods that fit into this category—cranberries and strawberries we already discussed, and then there are apples, raspberries, radishes, and more. But I'm limiting myself to sweet red peppers and tomatoes. However, keep in mind that because all of these foods share their red color, they also share many of the same nutrients, meaning they could offer similar health benefits.

Red Peppers

For starters, red peppers are loaded with vitamin C. When we think of the C vitamin, also called ascorbic acid, we often think oranges. But believe it or not, one medium red bell pepper has three times the vitamin C as one medium orange. Vitamin C helps to make *collagen*. Therefore it's important for making skin, tendons, ligaments, and bone. In addition, vitamin C is critical for proper wound healing. Its antioxidative powers protect us from the damage done by free radicals.

def•i•ni•tion

> **Collagen** is a protein that helps build connective tissue in your body.

Nutrition Information for ¹/₂ Cup of Red Peppers

Calories	20
Total Fat	0 grams
Saturated Fat	0 grams
Trans Fat	0 grams
Cholesterol	0 milligrams
Sodium	0 milligrams
Total Carbohydrate	4 grams
Dietary Fiber	1 gram
Sugars	3 grams
Protein	1 gram
Vitamin A	25% Daily Value
Vitamin C	240% Daily Value
Iron	2% Daily Value

In fact, vitamin C is so beneficial in repairing environmental damage to your body that it is the only vitamin with a higher *Recommended Daily Allowance* (*RDA*) for smokers. This is due to the extra cellular stress that smokers exert on their bodies.

def•i•ni•tion

The **Recommended Daily Allowance** or **RDA,** also called the recommended dietary allowance, is the amount of an essential nutrient, such as a vitamin or mineral, most healthy people need for adequate growth. RDAs are established by the National Academy of Sciences and were first developed in 1941.

Another antioxidant vitamin, vitamin A, is packed into red peppers as well. In fact, one medium pepper contains more than 100 percent of the RDA for vitamin A. This is a fat-soluble vitamin, which means it is stored in your body's fat. For that reason, it is possible to get too much; therefore megadose supplements of vitamin A or the other fat-soluble vitamins (D, E, and K) are not recommended.

A couple of vitamin A's key roles involve vision and reproduction health. It also helps to maintain the health of the surface linings of your eyes and respiratory, urinary, and intestinal tracts. These linings prevent bacteria and viruses from entering your body. By helping prevent the breakdown of the linings' tissue, vitamin A protects you from sickness.

In addition to vitamin A itself, red peppers contain *beta-carotene.*

def•i•ni•tion

> **Beta-carotene** is an antioxidant that is turned into vitamin A by the body. Among the several antioxidants that do this, beta-carotene is the easiest for the body to transform.

Okay, you know the drill by now. Antioxidants fight free radicals in your body to prevent the damage they do. As an antioxidant, that's just what beta-carotene does. Diets high in vitamin A and beta-carotene-rich foods appear to be linked with a lower risk of several types of cancer. One specific type is lung cancer. Eating a variety of foods containing high levels of these nutrients, such as red peppers, may help to decrease your risk of lung cancer.

Tomatoes

For a long time, tomatoes didn't really get much respect. They were just something you tossed into a salad or made into sauce for your pasta. I mean, how could something that's mostly juice and so incredibly low in calories have much in the way of nutrition?

Nutrition Information for One Medium Tomato

Calories	35
Total Fat	0.5 grams
Saturated Fat	0 grams
Trans Fat	0 grams
Cholesterol	0 milligrams
Sodium	5 milligrams
Total Carbohydrate	7 grams
Dietary Fiber	1 gram
Sugars	4 grams
Protein	1 gram
Vitamin A	20% Daily Value
Vitamin C	40% Daily Value
Calcium	2% Daily Value
Iron	2% Daily Value

Then researchers found there's more to good nutrition than just vitamins and minerals. The terms phytochemicals and antioxidants began popping up everywhere you turned. And wouldn't you know it, just like the other fruits and veggies, tomatoes have those powerful disease fighters, too. Turns out tomatoes and tomato products such as pasta and pizza sauce, and ketchup—yes I said pizza sauce and ketchup in a book about superfoods—are the best food sources of lycopene, an antioxidant in the carotenoid group of phytochemicals.

Kryptonite

Remember, this book is about super-*foods*, not super*pills*. Many of the health benefits I describe come from eating a variety of these foods. Vitamin and mineral supplements may not produce the same results. In fact, in the case of beta-carotene, supplements have been linked to an increased risk of lung cancer as well as death from lung cancer. What's that mean for you? Go ahead and eat all the red peppers and other vitamin A and beta-carotene-rich foods you like to obtain the numerous health benefits, but avoid taking beta-carotene supplements.

Lycopene's big claim to fame is the role it plays in decreasing the risk of prostate cancer. Lycopene has been shown to be an extremely powerful antioxidant. Eating tomatoes and tomato products regularly, at least twice a week as indicated by some research, may put you at a decreased risk for developing prostate cancer. In addition, frequent consumption of lycopene may also help treat prostate cancer by preventing it from spreading and keeping tumors smaller, according to one study.

Now before you ladies skip over this part, know that lycopene is such a powerful antioxidant that it can help you, too. It may reduce your likelihood of developing lung, breast, and stomach cancers. And it may play a role in cardiovascular health.

Still on the horizon for lycopene is skin protection from the sun's rays. Recent studies demonstrate that the inclusion of carotenoids, especially lycopene, in your diet may protect you from the damage done by ultraviolet light. This includes sunburn and could include skin cancer. By no means, however, should you consider eating tomatoes a substitute for using sunscreen when it comes to adequate sun protection. Continue to use sunscreen whenever you're in the sun's light.

Great Greens

Your mom probably said it, as did her mom, and hers before that—"Eat your greens." Turns out they knew of what they spoke. Green veggies, especially the dark-green leafy ones, are loaded with nutritional muscle.

Like the red peppers discussed earlier, dark-green veggies such as broccoli and spinach contain beta-carotene. So we know this compound in these vegetables helps decrease your risk of certain cancers, especially lung cancer.

In addition, another carotenoid called *lutein* is found in dark-green vegetables.

def•i•ni•tion

> **Lutein** is a carotenoid whose antioxidant powers work to benefit the eyes and heart as well as help prevent cancer.

In the body, high levels of lutein are found in the macula of the eye. Eating foods high in lutein may help prevent and slow macular degeneration, which is the leading cause of blindness in elderly men and women. The macula is special eye tissue that helps tell your brain what your eye is seeing. It is responsible for central vision, which enables you to drive and read as well as any other activity needing clear, straight-ahead vision. If the macula degenerates, this type of vision begins to deteriorate, leading to blindness.

Lutein also acts like an antioxidant in the eye by helping decrease the free-radical damage to the macula. In doing so, it helps prevent the development of cataracts.

Like many other antioxidants, lutein also plays a role in preventing heart disease. And we can't forget, like all vegetables, the dark-green ones are good sources of fiber, which can help lower blood cholesterol levels and prevent or improve constipation problems.

Another vitamin dark-green veggies are loaded with is vitamin K. Vitamin K's major role is initiating and regulating blood clotting. Without it, a simple little cut would cause you to lose as much blood as a major wound.

Kryptonite

Frequently when someone is prescribed the medications coumadin or warfarin, the person is told not to eat dark-green veggies. This is because these medications are blood thinners and eating large amounts of vitamin K could interfere in their work. However, there's no need to avoid these foods altogether. As long as you eat a consistent amount each day, your doctor can regulate your medication level based on that amount of dietary vitamin K.

Broccoli

President Bush (senior, that is) may hate the stuff, but boy is he missing out.

Nutrition Information for ½ Cup of Steamed Broccoli

Calories	20
Total Fat	0 grams
Saturated Fat	0 grams
Trans Fat	0 grams
Cholesterol	0 milligrams
Sodium	20 milligrams

continues

Nutrition Information for ¹/₂ Cup of Steamed Broccoli   (continued)

Total Carbohydrate	4 grams
Dietary Fiber	2 grams
Sugars	2 grams
Protein	2 grams
Vitamin A	25% Daily Value
Vitamin C	100% Daily Value
Calcium	4% Daily Value
Iron	4% Daily Value

Broccoli—along with other cruciferous vegetables such as cauliflower, brussels sprouts, kale, and cabbage—contains two unique phytochemicals called *indoles* and *isothiocyanates*. More research has been done with isothiocyanates, so I'm going to focus on them. One in particular, called *sulforaphane*, performs not just one but three different healthful jobs for us.

def•i•ni•tion

Indoles and **isothiocyanates** are anticancer property-containing phytochemicals found in cruciferous vegetables.

Sulforaphane is an isothiocyanate found in broccoli and broccoli sprouts.

Sulforaphane is a chemical found largely in broccoli and especially in broccoli sprouts. It's been shown to be very beneficial at slowing the growth of cancer cells and tumors. Studies have also shown that it increases cancer cell death. Both of these results are important when it comes to helping prevent cancer.

Affecting cancer cells isn't sulforaphane's only job. It's a great multitasker. This little phytochemical puts on hat number two to protect your eyes. The retina of your eyes is very sensitive to damaging oxidants. Ultraviolet rays from the sun is one of those oxidants that can do damage and lead to age-related macular degeneration and possibly blindness.

And job number three involves that nasty little H. pylori. H. pylori is the bacterium that causes the majority of stomach ulcers as well as a condition called gastritis. And in addition to the problems associated with gastritis itself, having it greatly increases your risk of stomach cancer. And it turns out that sulforaphane kills H. pylori. So in addition to the damage sulforaphane does to cancer cells in general, it plays a major role in helping prevent stomach cancer specifically.

Broccoli also contains the phytonutrient quercetin. If you remember from Chapter 2, this flavonoid appears to decrease the risk of developing asthma and lung cancer.

You can see how broccoli and even broccoli sprouts work throughout your body to both improve health and prevent disease.

Kryptonite

How you cook your veggies plays a big part in how many of these powerful nutrients you actually eat. Boiling and microwaving vegetables in water can lead to losses of up to 97 percent of the key antioxidants. Whenever possible, stick to steaming them over water, which will retain 89 to 100 percent of the vitamins, minerals, and other nutrients.

Spinach

Who among us can't recall an image of Popeye's muscles bulging after he inhaled spinach from a can? Well, it may not exactly do that for you and me, but it still does our bodies good.

Nutrition Information for 1 Cup of Raw Spinach

Calories	5
Total Fat	0.5 grams
Saturated Fat	0 grams
Trans Fat	0 grams
Cholesterol	0 milligrams
Sodium	25 milligrams
Total Carbohydrate	1 gram
Dietary Fiber	1 gram
Sugars	0 grams

Protein	1 gram
Vitamin A	60% Daily Value
Vitamin C	15% Daily Value
Calcium	2% Daily Value
Iron	4% Daily Value

One thing to take note of with spinach is the apparent tremendous difference in nutrient content between raw and cooked. It would seem that cooked spinach is far more nutritious. In reality the two are quite similar ounce for ounce. When cooked, however, spinach wilts down to less than one sixth of its original size. Therefore, eating a little more than 3 cups of raw spinach gives you the same nutrition as one half cup of cooked spinach. But keep in mind what I said earlier about cooking vegetables. To preserve nutrients, you shouldn't cook the life out of your leafy greens, just steam them over a small amount of water until they wilt down. Also, I am by no means saying that raw spinach isn't nutritious. It is very much so. I'm just saying cooked spinach is a more concentrated nutrient source.

Nutrition Information for ¹/₂ Cup of Steamed Spinach

Calories	20
Total Fat	0 grams
Saturated Fat	0 grams
Trans Fat	0 grams

continues

Nutrition Information for $\frac{1}{2}$ Cup of Steamed Spinach (continued)

Cholesterol	0 milligrams
Sodium	65 milligrams
Total Carbohydrate	3 grams
Dietary Fiber	2 grams
Sugars	0 grams
Protein	3 grams
Vitamin A	190% Daily Value
Vitamin C	15% Daily Value
Calcium	10% Daily Value
Iron	20% Daily Value

A newly found bonus from leafy spinach is its high magnesium content. Magnesium is one of the minerals our body uses for any number of functions. Scientists recently identified a link between magnesium intake and the risk of *metabolic syndrome*.

def•i•ni•tion

Metabolic syndrome is a group of risk factors linked to heart disease and diabetes. The risk factors include high blood pressure, low HDL cholesterol, high blood sugar, high triglycerides (the major form of fat), and abdominal fat.

Researchers determined that people eating magnesium-rich diets were much less likely to develop cardiovascular disease and diabetes than those whose magnesium intake was low. They've not yet determined the daily intake amount necessary to achieve such benefits. However, with its 78 milligrams, one half cup of cooked spinach contains almost one quarter of the current RDA of 300–400 milligrams.

Kryptonite

If you tend to use a lot of low-fat and fat-free foods, especially products like salad dressings that you would eat with veggies, take note. While veggies are fat-free, many of the nutrients in them, such as beta-carotene, need fat to be absorbed and used by our bodies. By pouring some fat-free dressing onto a bowl full of nutrient-packed veggies or dipping your baby carrots into some fat-free dip, you're not getting as much nutrient power as you could be. To maximize your nutrition quotient, drizzle some healthy olive oil over your bunch of greens and go ahead and munch those carrots with some full-fat or low-fat dip.

Believe it or not, spinach has something in common with blueberries. Who would've guessed that? They both contain the flavonol myricetin. More work with humans needs to be investigated about this nutrient, but early information is promising. Myricetin appears to have both anti-inflammatory and anti-cancer properties, which means it may be beneficial in preventing and improving not only cancer but also heart disease and inflammatory diseases such as arthritis. In addition, myricetin might play a role in transporting sugar from the blood into fat cells, and therefore might be involved in treating diabetes. But again, more studies with humans must be done to confirm these big benefits.

Super Knowledge

Two other minerals are found in high amounts in spinach but don't pack quite the same nutritional punch. Spinach is high in both iron and calcium. One half cup of cooked spinach contains about the same amount of calcium as one half cup of milk. But (yes, there's a but) spinach also contains compounds called oxalates, which bind with both iron and calcium before they can be absorbed and work their wonders on you. So while you may see lists including spinach as a good source of these two minerals, keep in mind it's not as helpful in this area as other foods, such as meat and chicken (for iron) and low-fat dairy foods (for calcium).

Spinach plays double duty when it comes to helping your eyes. It contains lutein, which as I said earlier helps maintain eye health. It also contains lutein's partner in crime, zeaxanthin. Zeaxanthin is a carotenoid that works as an antioxidant, protecting the eye and preventing certain cancers. It's found in green leafy vegetables and yellow and orange fruits and vegetables.

Just like lutein, zeaxanthin helps to maintain good vision by keeping the macula of the eye healthy. It protects the eye from damage that can cause age-related macular degeneration as well as cataracts.

Outstanding Oranges

This section's a bit like that movie, *Four Weddings and a Funeral*, except we've got three vegetables and a fruit. You're probably thinking, sure, carrots and sweet potatoes and pumpkin, they probably have a lot in common, but oranges? What is she thinking?

Believe it or not, while they each have their own special traits, they do share common properties, the reason being that they share a common color. You may have figured this out by now, that the components giving fruits and veggies their brilliant colors are the same ones giving them their super health powers.

One nutrient this mix of fruit and veggies has is beta-cryptoxanthin, another of the carotenoids that the body converts to vitamin A.

Beta-cryptoxanthin is similar to beta-carotene but not quite as powerful. It contains about half the vitamin A power of beta-carotene, which is the major vitamin A precursor. Due to its association with vitamin A, this phytochemical is important in maintaining eye health and vision, boosting your immune system, and keeping your skin and bones healthy. One unique property of this phytonutrient seems to be its role in helping prevent the painful condition arthritis.

As if it weren't enough to have a powerful vitamin A precursor in these yummy foods, it turns out they also contain the most powerful one. That's right, these orange-colored parts of nature's feast are loaded with beta-carotene itself. So just go ahead and double most of the benefits I mentioned for beta-cryptoxanthin when you chow down on these guys.

Sweet Potatoes

For a few of us, perhaps the only time we eat sweet potatoes is when they're covered in gooey marshmallows and placed next to some roasted turkey. I'm here to tell you that's just not enough!

Nutrition Information for One Medium Baked Sweet Potato

Calories	100
Total Fat	0 grams
Saturated Fat	0 grams
Trans Fat	0 grams
Cholesterol	0 milligrams
Sodium	40 milligrams

Total Carbohydrate	24 grams
Dietary Fiber	4 grams
Sugars	10 grams
Protein	2 grams
Vitamin A	440% Daily Value
Vitamin C	35% Daily Value
Calcium	4% Daily Value
Iron	4% Daily Value

Of the orange produce, sweet potatoes don't have much beta-cryptoxanthin, but boy are they loaded with beta-carotene! There isn't an RDA for beta-carotene, but based on vitamin A requirements, you could actually meet your body's needs by eating just one medium sweet potato. While it can be harmful to consume excessive amounts of vitamin A, that's not the case with beta-carotene. The body will convert as much as it needs to and will excrete the rest. So go ahead and eat sweet potatoes and other orange veggies to your heart's content. If you do eat large amounts of beta-carotene, you may notice your palms and the soles of your feet turn pale orange, but this isn't harmful and the normal color returns once your beta-carotene intake decreases.

One of beta-carotene's big jobs is keeping your eyes healthy and your vision good. It's a key component in helping prevent age-related macular degeneration, the leading cause of preventable blindness in developed countries.

I hope you agree that serving this vegetable more than once a year is certainly worth it. Both baking and roasting it bring out the natural sweetness while preserving the nutrients that boiling could remove.

Kryptonite

It's important to note that to gain many, if not all, of the benefits discussed in this book, you must obtain these nutrients from a varied diet of whole foods, not from a pill out of a bottle. It can be easy to overdose when taking supplements, as they often contain 100 percent or more of the RDA for many nutrients. And more is not always better—in some instances it can be dangerous. In addition, healthy foods are rich in a variety of vitamins, minerals, and other nutrients. Oftentimes the synergy between the naturally occurring components helps to produce or magnify the benefits. This synergy can't be replicated in a bottle.

The Great Pumpkin

Charlie Brown's pal Linus may have been hoping for candy, but little did he know how great the pumpkin really is.

Nutrition Information for ½ Cup of Puréed Pumpkin

Calories	40
Total Fat	0 grams
Saturated Fat	0 grams
Trans Fat	0 grams
Cholesterol	0 milligrams
Sodium	5 milligrams
Total Carbohydrate	10 grams
Dietary Fiber	4 grams
Sugars	4 grams
Protein	1 gram
Vitamin A	380% Daily Value
Vitamin C	8% Daily Value
Calcium	4% Daily Value
Iron	10% Daily Value

Time to meet a new carotene. Alpha-carotene, yet another carotenoid and precursor to vitamin A, is found in high amounts in pumpkin.

Like the other carotenes, alpha is important for immune system functioning, healthy skin and bones, and vision. It also works as an antioxidant and therefore can be beneficial in lowering your risk of heart disease and certain cancers. In addition, as an antioxidant protecting body cells from damage, alpha-carotene may help slow the aging process.

Kryptonite

The ingredient Olestra, which is used as a fat substitute in low-fat potato chips and other snack foods, and the plant sterols in margarines such as Benecol and Take Control, may decrease the absorption of carotenoids like alpha- and beta-carotene. If these foods are part of your regular diet, be sure that at least some of the times you eat carotenoid-rich foods, you do so at a different time than you eat these chips or margarines.

As I said in Chapter 2, often frozen and canned fruits and veggies are just as nutritious as fresh (if not more so). Fortunately that's the case with pumpkin, too. It's a whole lot easier to open up a can of puréed pumpkin than it is to open, seed, cut, roast, and mash a fresh pumpkin. Besides, canned pumpkin is available year-round. Just be sure to get plain pumpkin, not the pumpkin-pie mix.

Not sure what do to with pumpkin? You're not alone. Many of us aren't sure what to with it besides baking it with a few other ingredients in a pie crust and topping with whipped cream. You can use pumpkin in place of mashed sweet potatoes in a casserole. And you can mix a can of pumpkin purée with any flavor of box cake mix instead of the oil, eggs, and water. And certainly go ahead and make that pie filling, but skip the crust, where most of the fat comes from, for a healthy dessert. You can also use it like bananas in quick breads or muffins.

Carrots

They may not look as good on your finger as a gold ring, but carrots sure help your insides look good.

Nutrition Information for 1/2 Cup of Cooked Carrots

Calories	25
Total Fat	0 grams
Saturated Fat	0 grams
Trans Fat	0 grams
Cholesterol	0 milligrams
Sodium	45 milligrams
Total Carbohydrate	6 grams
Dietary Fiber	2 grams
Sugars	3 grams
Protein	1 gram
Vitamin A	270% Daily Value
Vitamin C	4% Daily Value
Calcium	2% Daily Value
Iron	2% Daily Value

Like the other colorful veggies, carrots are packed full of carotenoids such as beta- and alpha-carotene. In fact, just 1 cup contains more than 250 percent of the suggested daily needs, as well as almost 700 percent of the RDA for vitamin A. Wow!

It's those antioxidants that help to make carrots powerful disease fighters. Studies suggest that people who eat on average at least one serving of carrots a day dramatically reduced their risk of having a heart attack compared to people who eat less than one serving per day.

And when it comes to cancer, people with high intakes of carotenoids have been shown to cut their risk of postmenopausal breast cancer by 20 percent. Eating foods with high carotenoid content has also been shown to result in an up to 50 percent decrease in the occurrence of bladder, cervical, prostate, colon, larynx, and esophageal cancers. And the unique carotenoid and phytochemical combination found in carrots, including alpha-carotene, appears to be protective against lung cancer as well.

Recent research has begun looking into the role that carotenoids may play in diabetes. It seems that high blood levels of carotenoids may assist in lowering blood sugar levels and decreasing the likelihood of developing diabetes. However, much more research needs to be done regarding this connection with specific fruits and vegetables.

Oranges

They may seem like misfits in a vegetable chapter, but nutritionally speaking, oranges fit right in.

Nutrition Information for One Medium Orange

Calories	70
Total Fat	0 grams
Saturated Fat	0 grams
Trans Fat	0 grams
Cholesterol	0 milligrams
Sodium	0 milligrams
Total Carbohydrate	21 grams
Dietary Fiber	7 grams
Sugars	14 grams
Protein	1 gram
Vitamin A	2% Daily Value
Vitamin C	130% Daily Value
Calcium	6% Daily Value
Iron	2% Daily Value

You may recall I've mentioned other foods containing more vitamin C than oranges, but as C is the orange's claim to fame, I've saved the detailed description of all of its benefits for now. After all, one orange does have more than the RDA for vitamin C.

First you should know that vitamin C is a water-soluble vitamin. A benefit to being water-soluble is that your body doesn't store it. In other words, if you eat more than you need, your body simply excretes it. In fact, you can safely eat up to 2,000 milligrams a day without problems.

Vitamin C is needed for the growth and repair of your body tissue and for the formation of collagen. Therefore it's essential for helping wounds to heal properly and repairing and maintaining things like cartilage, bones, and teeth.

As another powerful antioxidant, vitamin C helps combat the free radicals responsible for aging, and those that play a factor in the development of cancer, heart disease, and arthritis. In addition, vitamin C and other antioxidants protect your body from external toxins like cigarette smoke, pollution, and chemicals.

Another big bonus vitamin C gives you is that it helps your body absorb *iron* from your food.

def•i•ni•tion

> **Iron** is a mineral that is essential to obtain from your diet. It's used to make hemoglobin, which is the component in blood that carries oxygen throughout the body to where it's needed.

Without adequate iron, you could develop iron-deficient anemia, the most common nutritional deficiency in the world. Vitamin C helps your body maximize the iron you consume from foods like meat, chicken, eggs, and fortified cereals. For this to happen, the vitamin C and the iron must be eaten at the same time. So enjoy a few juicy orange slices with your iron-fortified breakfast cereal, or stir-fry some red peppers to have with your grilled steak.

And we can't forget the common cold. Vitamin C enhances the work of the immune system and may help protect us from illness.

But even the healthiest of us succumb to a cold every now and again. During infections or times of stress, your body uses more vitamin C. Therefore, ensuring an adequate regular intake is crucial to prepare for these times. In addition, when you're sick, extra vitamin C can help. Taking up to 1 gram a day may lessen the severity of your symptoms, as well as shorten the length of time you're sick. It may not be a cure, but any improvement sounds good to me. And remember, because your body doesn't store excessive amounts of vitamin C, you can feel comfortable kicking up your intake a bit when you're under the weather.

Oranges also contain phytochemicals called flavanones (a type of flavonoid), specifically *hesperetin* and *naringenin*.

def•i•ni•tion

Hesperetin and **naringenin** are flavonoids shown in animal studies to possess many health-promoting properties involving blood pressure, inflammation, and heart disease.

More work in humans is still on the horizon for these two compounds; however, they have shown some promise. Higher intakes of both of these nutrients have been associated with a decreased incidence of both strokes and asthma.

The Rest of the Rainbow

So you've heard about reds and greens and oranges, but what about the rest? When you were young, you may have learned the acronym ROY G BIV to help you remember the colors of the rainbow. I've covered three, but there are still other important colors growing out of our gardens. In addition, within each color group, I've discussed just a few foods. You should know that there are more than 100 fruits and vegetables you can choose from every day to eat your rainbow and reap the health benefits.

Here are a few nutritious examples from each color group I didn't discuss, as well as more examples from the three groups I did include.

Red

- Red apples
- Red grapes
- Raspberries
- Watermelon
- Beets
- Red potatoes
- Red onions
- Radishes

Orange/Yellow

- Cantaloupe
- Grapefruit

- Mangoes
- Pineapple
- Butternut squash
- Yellow peppers
- Yellow summer squash

Green

- Avocados
- Green grapes
- Kiwifruit
- Asparagus
- Brussels sprouts
- Green beans
- Zucchini

Blue/Purple

- Blackberries
- Dried plums/prunes
- Plums
- Raisins
- Purple cabbage
- Eggplant

White

- Bananas
- White nectarines
- White peaches

- Cauliflower
- Garlic
- Onions
- Potatoes (white fleshed)

This is less than one third of the variety of choices you have each and every day to live healthier. So go on and color your plate with health.

The Least You Need to Know

- Vegetables, especially the brightly or deeply colored ones, are an extremely low-calorie and fiber-filled source of a variety of powerful, disease-fighting nutrients.
- To obtain the greatest health benefits, be sure to eat a variety of fruits and vegetables from each color group every day.
- Steaming vegetables will not only maintain their vibrant colors but also their powerful vitamins, minerals, and other nutrients.
- Vitamin C can be found in a variety of fruits and veggies, not just oranges.

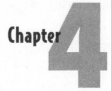

Chapter 4

Drink to Your Health

In This Chapter

- Not only are there superfoods but there are superdrinks, too
- Grape juice isn't just for kids
- Enjoying a glass of wine with dinner isn't a bad thing
- Antioxidants aren't found only in fruits and vegetables

So far I've talked only about foods, but many drinks are beneficial to your health as well. Some are loaded with vitamins and minerals, while others possess those power-filled phytochemicals. Most, however, include a combination of these health-promoting and disease-fighting nutrients.

Grape Juice

Who'd have known that the drink you loved as a kid was not just great-tasting but so great for you?

When it comes to grape juice, there are two different kinds: purple and white. And we're not just talking about any grape juice. No, we're talking about juice made from specific grapes. To obtain the health benefits from purple grapes, be sure to drink juice made from Concord grapes. Usually the juice is called Concord grape juice. And when it comes to white grape juice, the word to remember is Niagara.

These types of grapes both have thick skins and seeds. These are the parts of the grapes that contain most of the health-assisting phytochemicals. Some grape juices are made with seedless grapes. While they make great easy snacks, they don't make a juice with nearly the nutrient wallop as juices made from Concord and Niagara grapes. So be sure to check the label and/or the ingredients list when you're buying what could become your new favorite drink.

Purple Concord Grape Juice

It may be a mess to clean up when you spill it, but the work it does on your insides is far from a mess.

Nutrition Information for 1 Cup (8 fl. oz.) of Concord Grape Juice

Calories	170
Total Fat	0 grams
Saturated Fat	0 grams

Trans Fat	0 grams
Cholesterol	0 milligrams
Sodium	20 milligrams
Total Carbohydrate	42 grams
Dietary Fiber	0 grams
Sugars	40 grams
Protein	0 grams
Vitamin C	100% Daily Value

Concord grape juice contributes to heart health in a number of ways. Of course that deep purple color signifies that it holds powerful antioxidant activity. The flavonoids in Concord grape juice slow the oxidation of LDL or "bad" cholesterol. LDLs circulate in the bloodstream, attach to the inner walls of your arteries for a while, and then go into the bloodstream again. While they are attached to the artery walls, they are likely to oxidate. Oxidation during this time leads to *atherosclerosis*. By slowing this oxidation, flavonoids make it less likely it will occur when the LDLs are attached to the artery walls; by doing so, they decrease the progression of heart disease.

def•i•ni•tion

Atherosclerosis is thickening and hardening of artery walls due to fat deposits on their lining. It's responsible for a great deal of coronary artery/heart disease as well as strokes.

Besides being an antioxidant, purple Concord grape juice has many other avenues in which it benefits your health. Nitric oxide (NO) is a compound that plays a role in maintaining a healthy cardiovascular system. Properties in the juice increase the production of NO and thus improve your heart health. NO levels in both the blood and the endothelium (the inside lining of the artery walls) are increased by Concord grape juice.

The endothelial NO improves the flexibility of your arterial walls. This is important because supple arteries are easily expanded, allowing for greater blood supply to get to where it needs to, when it needs to.

According to researchers, Concord grape juice acts similarly to aspirin when it comes to protecting your heart. It appears to inhibit the inclination of blood platelets to stick together and form blood clots. When pieces of blood clots break off and begin to circulate through the arteries, they can lodge in dangerous places and lead to heart attacks and strokes. Preventing the formation of clots in the first place is a big step to preventing the crippling, and many times deadly, problems associated with them.

If all Concord grape juice did was help our hearts, it'd be well worth drinking. But there's more. Like the antioxidants in some of the other fruits and vegetables, those found in Concord grape juice may play a role in cancer protection. Research is still in the preliminary stages, but it's been shown that Concord grape juice could reduce the growth of breast cancer cells in more than one of the stages of the disease's development.

And finally, one more area of health improvement that helps Concord grape juice claim its superfood status. This, too, is still in the early point of its research. Concord grape juice may help improve two of the negative issues associated with the aging process. It appears that drinking the juice regularly could improve short-term memory. Including Concord grape juice in your usual diet may also improve motor function. That is the ability to perform both large and small body movements such as walking, sitting, and picking things up with your hands.

Before you start thinking you have to drink a gallon of juice a day to reap the benefits, let me correct you. The research done so far has produced results with only about 9 to 11 ounces per day. That's just over a cup—not too much at all.

White Niagara Grape Juice

It may be lacking the deep purple color, but white grape juice made from Niagara grapes still has plenty of health benefits.

Nutrition Information for 1 Cup (8 fl. oz.) of Niagara Grape Juice

Calories	160
Total Fat	0 grams
Saturated Fat	0 grams

continues

Nutrition Information for 1 Cup (8 fl. oz.) of Niagara Grape Juice (continued)

Trans Fat	0 grams
Cholesterol	0 milligrams
Sodium	20 milligrams
Total Carbohydrate	39 grams
Sugars	37 grams
Protein	0 grams
Vitamin C	100% Daily Value

While white grape juice possesses benefits for people of all ages, it's most helpful for infants and toddlers. Babies still developing digestive systems can't handle many of the foods and drinks we as adults consume daily. Components in some fruit juices can be problematic, as can unequal amounts of different carbohydrates. Sorbitol, a natural sugar alcohol, as well as containing more *fructose* than *glucose*, can cause carbohydrate-absorption problems in babies. This malabsorption contributes to the symptoms many babies experience when drinking some fruit juices. The symptoms can include gas, bloating, discomfort, crying, diarrhea, and difficulty sleeping after eating. White grape juice does not contain sorbitol but does contain an equal balance of carbohydrates. For these reasons, infants drinking white grape juice do not tend to suffer the uncomfortable problems associated with some other juices.

def•i•ni•tion

Fructose is a sugar found naturally in fruits.
Glucose is the sugar that is our body's
main source of energy.

When young children have infections affecting
their digestive systems, their gastrointestinal tract
is even more sensitive to the sugars in juices. It's
been shown that white grape juice is better tolerated than other juices by infants and toddlers after
a case of diarrhea, resulting in fewer messy diapers.

Kryptonite

Because too much juice can fill young
children's little tummies and make them
less hungry for other nutritious foods and
drinks, the American Academy of Pediatrics
has set guidelines. Serve only 100 percent
fruit juice to kids of all ages, and limit 1- to
6-year-olds to 4–6 ounces per day, and
limit 7- to 18-year-olds to no more than
8–12 ounces per day.

Just because you're all grown up doesn't mean
you have to trade in your white grape juice for
something else. 100 percent grape juice made with
Niagara grapes has more antioxidant power than
more than 50 other clear 100 percent fruit juices.
In fact, in laboratory tests, it was shown to have
more antioxidant capacity than all juices except for

purple Concord grape juice and grapefruit juice.
This is because Niagara grapes are loaded with
those powerful antioxidant flavonoids. These phytochemicals in white Niagara grape juice help to
protect you from heart disease and certain cancers.

Red Wine

You may have heard that red wine is good for you,
but do you really know how good?

Nutrition Information for 4 Fluid Ounces of Red Wine

Calories	100
Total Fat	0 grams
Saturated Fat	0 grams
Trans Fat	0 grams
Cholesterol	0 milligrams
Sodium	0 milligrams
Total Carbohydrate	3 grams
Fiber	0 grams
Sugars	1 gram
Protein	0 grams
Iron	4% Daily Value

Red wine has received the most notoriety for con-
tributing to heart health and it does so in a number

of ways. Because it's made from grapes, it contains many phytochemicals like other fruits and veggies. In fact, you may notice that red wine produces many similar benefits to grape juice. However, there are some benefits unique to red wine. Because red wine is made by letting the grapes' skins and seeds ferment in the grapes' juices, and those are the parts where the majority of phytochemicals are found, red wine has very high levels of these powerhouses. White wine also contains some but not nearly as much, because the skins and seeds are removed early in the white-wine-making process.

One of the key components in red wine is *resveratrol*. Resveratrol is considered a phytoestrogen. This means that it has similar properties to the female sex hormone estrogen. Therefore it's able to act like estrogen in the body and may offer benefits for certain conditions affected by decreases in natural estrogen such as menopause, breast cancer, osteoporosis, and heart disease.

def•i•ni•tion

Resveratrol is an antioxidant found in high amounts in red wine, grapes, raspberries, and peanuts.

To improve your heart's health, red wine takes many approaches. Resveratrol is responsible for more than one. First, it decreases the oxidation of the bad cholesterol, LDL. If you remember, that means it helps prevent the damage done by free radicals caused by both external and internal toxins. By doing so, it slows the progression of heart disease.

Resveratrol also helps prevent blood cells from sticking together. This means that they can't bunch up together as easily to form dangerous blood clots that could cut off the oxygen supply to important organs. A blood clot blockage in a vessel in the heart can cause a heart attack; one in the brain can cause a stroke.

Another way resveratrol benefits heart health involves nitric oxide. If you recall, this is a substance that helps blood flow more easily by letting your blood vessels relax. In doing so, it enables blood to get to where it's needed quickly. One study showed that this particular action may help to prevent future heart attacks in men who've already had a heart attack. Improved blood flow could offer the benefit of helping prevent a stroke as well.

Along with resveratrol there's another antioxidant found in red wine, saponin. This is one of those benefits that makes red wine stand out. Saponin may help decrease blood levels of LDL cholesterol. That's right, something that finally helps to get rid of that bad guy. Lower levels of LDL mean less plaque can build up within your arteries and signify a lower risk of having a heart attack. Red wine also helps to boost your HDL or good cholesterol levels. Increased HDL levels are yet another significant factor in decreasing your risk of heart disease.

Kryptonite

If you're not a drinker, don't feel you must become one to achieve health benefits. Many, many benefits can be obtained from a diet rich in a variety of the other foods and drinks I discuss in this book. While red wine offers many health benefits, too much can be harmful, and it's not for everyone. Women who are pregnant or trying to conceive shouldn't drink alcohol due to potential birth defects. Those with a history or strong family history of alcohol problems may choose to avoid alcohol. You shouldn't drive while under the influence of alcohol. And be aware that alcohol does not safely mix with certain medications. If you're unsure, speak to your doctor.

In addition to the heart benefits, red wine may play a role in cancer prevention. And guess what? That ole resveratrol is back. It may be beneficial in regard to several types of cancers. Studies show that it inhibits the growth and spread of cancer. It does so by preventing the production of new blood vessels needed to feed the tumors. By doing so, resveratrol cuts off the nutrient supply, and therefore limits the growth of the tumors.

But more than that, resveratrol makes certain cancer cells destroy themselves. So far this self-destruction of cancer cells has been seen in breast cancer, skin cancer, and leukemia cells.

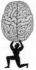

Super Knowledge

Does it matter what kind of wine you drink? It just might. Turns out that cabernet sauvignon contains the greatest amount of flavonoids. Petit syrah and pinot noir run a close second, and merlots and red zinfandels contain the least.

So how many times a day should you be saying "Cheers!"? More research is needed for a definitive answer to this question, partly due to the fact that antioxidant amount in wine varies depending on the types of grapes, as well as how and when they were grown. But one serving of wine is a 4-ounce glass. The recommendations at this point are one to two servings for men and one serving for women per day. These amounts will maximize the health benefits while providing the least amount of problems associated with heavier drinking. Studies show that people drinking three or more alcoholic beverages per day are at an increased risk for high blood pressure and high triglycerides—a fat found in the blood.

Tea

Did you know that tea is the second most commonly consumed beverage in the world, behind water?

Nutrition Information for 8 Fluid Ounces of Unsweetened Tea

Calories	0
Total Fat	0 grams
Saturated Fat	0 grams
Trans Fat	0 grams
Cholesterol	0 milligrams
Sodium	5 milligrams
Total Carbohydrate	1 gram
Fiber	0 grams
Sugars	0 grams
Protein	0 grams

So what is it all these tea drinkers know that the rest of us don't? Because of its high antioxidant content, tea has been shown to play a role in preventing many diseases and health conditions. That's right, tea is full of those darn antioxidants, too!

Kryptonite

The type of tea that has been studied for its health benefits is from the camellia sinensis plant. This includes black, green, oolong, and white tea. Herbal teas are not from the same plant and so while they may also have health benefits, they've not been studied to the same extent and are not included in this book.

The primary beneficial flavonoids found in tea are flavanols and flavonols. Specifically, the flavanols tea contains are catechins, theaflavins, and thearubigins. And the flavonols are quercetin, kaempferol, myricetin, and isorhamnetin.

With regard to the flavanols, how the tea is made is important. White and green teas are made with unfermented tea leaves. They contain high amounts of catechins but low amounts of theaflavins and thearubigins. Black tea, on the other hand, is made from fully fermented tea leaves. It's rich in theaflavins and thearubigins but does not contain much in the way of catechins. Finally, oolong tea is made from partially fermented leaves, and therefore the catechin, theaflavin, and thearubigin content is somewhere in between that of both black and white and green teas.

Even though the antioxidant content varies a bit among the different types of tea, they all contain about the same amount of antioxidant power. Studies done on the different teas have produced similar results when it comes to health benefits.

The most studied area with regard to tea and your health involves cancer protection. Tea has many lines of attack when it comes to cancer. The first is fighting the damage free radicals do that can lead to cancer development. Another is helping prevent uncontrolled cell growth, which is what leads to the growth and spread of the disease. Yet another is encouraging cancer cell death. And finally, tea heightens your immune system, increasing its ability to fight off the development and growth of cancer cells.

Not only does tea work in a multitude of ways to battle cancer, it also works on several different types of cancer. A number of studies have been conducted on both men and women with regard to tea-drinking and a variety of digestive cancers. The findings show that those who drink tea compared to those who don't had reduced risks of colon, rectal, and urinary tract cancers. These studies involved drinking between 1½ to 2½ cups of tea per day. An additional study demonstrates a lower risk of colon, rectal, and pancreatic cancer in those drinking 3 to 4½ cups of tea a day. And another showed a relationship between high tea-flavonoid intake and a lower risk of stomach cancer.

In terms of ovarian cancer, woman who drink the most tea are the least likely to develop the disease. In this study tea consumption was defined as at least 2 cups per day. However, drinking even 1 cup per day also reduced a woman's risk—just not as much.

Tea drinkers also appear to have a decreased risk of developing skin cancer. It's important to note that strength of the tea, brewing time, and temperature all seem to influence the protective benefits of tea against skin cancer. Also, drinking tea shouldn't be considered a replacement for proper sunscreen usage. Tea is also being investigated for the benefits it seems to offer against oral and lung cancers.

Tea's role in cardiovascular health has also been looked at a great deal. For the most part, studies show that 3 or more cups of tea per day is the amount needed to reduce your risk of heart disease and stroke. As with cancer, tea addresses heart health in a number of ways.

Drinking a couple of cups of tea a day appears to reduce the chances of having a heart attack as well as decrease the risk of dying from a heart attack if you do have one. This result was seen in both people who had had a heart attack and those who'd never had one.

Those drinking a couple of cups of tea per day also seem to have a reduced risk of developing high blood pressure compared to those drinking less tea. While a disease itself, high blood pressure also puts you at an increased risk of having a stroke or heart attack. And a recent study looked more closely at how tea performs all these wonders. It showed that by drinking tea regularly, people who already have cardiovascular disease can improve the health and performance of their blood vessels, allowing for better blood flow.

Regular tea drinkers may have lower total cholesterol, LDL cholesterol, and triglyceride levels than nontea drinkers, therefore lowering their risk of having a heart attack. These results, however, were found with drinking 5 or more cups of tea per day, not the 3 I mentioned above.

With all the cancer and heart protection benefits tea provides, there's still more! Drinking tea boosts the immune system to help you fight nasty infections from bacteria, viruses, and fungi. Tea flavonoids may also prevent bacteria in the mouth from forming plaque, which could mean fewer cavities.

And while doctors often recommend upping your fluid intake to help prevent kidney stones, apparently the type of fluid you choose to drink may be important. Studies have shown that for every 8-ounce cup of tea you drink, you could be lowering your likelihood of developing kidney stones by 8 to 14 percent.

Super Knowledge

A panel of medical and nutrition experts recently created the Healthy Beverage Guidelines. Beverages were ranked according to their nutrient density as well as scientific evidence that they provide either a health benefit or risk. Due to the fact that it's calorie-free but provides many health benefits, tea is ranked in the number two spot, second only to water. The panel recommends up to five 8-ounce servings of unsweetened tea per day.

The Least You Need to Know

- The kind of grapes used to make juice affects the antioxidant content.
- How wine is made is a determining factor of its nutritional power.
- Drinking tea offers health benefits from head to toe.
- Herbal teas may not offer the same health benefits as black, green, and oolong teas.

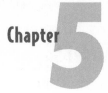

Soy and Yogurt

In This Chapter

- How soy can be part of your diet
- Isoflavones aren't a new flavor at Baskin-Robbins
- Bacteria isn't all bad
- Calcium—it's more than just a bone-builder

Thirty or so years ago, soybeans and yogurt were pretty much designated as hippie food—the foods on which health food stores thrived.

Who would've thought that a few years down the line there'd be so many different types of yogurt that it would fill as many shelves at the grocery store as the cheese section? Or that soy would be made into everything from milk to burgers and from cheese to bacon-flavored slices? Or that people would be snacking on soy nuts and edamame?

Soy and yogurt, as well as the foods and drinks made from them, could almost be considered staples of the American diet. It'd be tough to find a household without at least one of these foods or beverages.

Super Soy

Believe it or not, soybeans have been in humans' diets for thousands of years. Its versatility is probably part of the reason for that. Soy sauce and soybean oil, which is a common ingredient in mayonnaise and salad dressing, have been around for years. But other soy foods have started to achieve more widespread popularity just in the last decade or so.

Super Knowledge

Even though soybeans are a plant food, the protein found within them is similar to the protein found in animal products such as meat, milk, and eggs. It is a complete protein, meaning that it contains all the amino acids your body needs to grow and develop normally but cannot make by itself.

So how does soy work its wonders? Two components in soy are responsible for most of the health benefits. These are the protein and the *isoflavones*.

def•i•ni•tion

Isoflavones are compounds found in plants that mildly act like the reproductive hormone estrogen. They are also called phytoestrogens and are found in chickpeas and legumes, the soybean being the legume with the most.

These two elements are responsible for decreasing heart disease risk and menopause symptoms, and possibly preventing certain cancers. Just how much of these two items are in the different types of soy foods depends on the food itself. Whole soybean-based foods like tofu, soymilk, and soy flour contain the most protein and isoflavones. Soy protein concentrates may not contain many isoflavones due to processing. The foods they are found in, such as soy burgers and soy dogs, contain even less because they also contain many nonsoy ingredients. And lastly, because they contain no soy protein, soy sauce and soybean oil contain no isoflavones.

Now you know what they are and what they're in, so just what do these guys do? All sorts of good stuff, is the simple answer to that question.

The most studied benefit with the most proven research is soy's role in heart disease. When it comes to heart disease, soy works in a number of ways to decrease your cardiovascular risks. Soy protein itself can help lower your total cholesterol as well as your LDL cholesterol (often called "bad" cholesterol). In fact, soy protein in a diet including almonds and fiber has been shown to be just as effective as some cholesterol-lowering medications.

Soy's second job in heart-disease prevention involves isoflavones. The isoflavones found in soy protein may increase your levels of HDL cholesterol, or good cholesterol. Isoflavones also protect LDLs from oxidation. Oxidized LDL leads to the development of atherosclerosis or hardening of the arteries, which is an early sign of heart disease.

If you're a menopausal woman, or soon will be, and suffer from hot flashes, I've got some cool news for you. A daily dose of soy may just help decrease those annoying and uncomfortable power surges. This has been found in women eating a diet high in isoflavones, not just the protein.

While more research is needed, there is some evidence showing that daily consumption of soy protein with high levels of isoflavones may help to improve bone mass in the spine. This can help women suffering from or at high risk for *osteoporosis*.

def•i•ni•tion

> **Osteoporosis** is a disease in which your bones become less dense and more porous. This sometimes-painful condition increases your chances of fracturing bones and makes your hips and spine especially vulnerable. Osteoporosis can affect men as well as women, and while it can start even when you're young, the results are usually seen when you reach your sixties or after. So prevention, starting when you're a child, is the key.

Soy may also be involved in preventing certain types of cancer. This area is still a bit contradictory and studies are ongoing to iron out the details. The link between soy and cancer exists because of the way soy isoflavones weakly imitate hormonal functions. And the cancers involved are those with a hormonal component like breast and prostate.

Several research studies show that eating soy foods decreases the risk of breast cancer. This area became of interest when it was noticed that Asian women had some of the lowest rates of breast cancer compared to women of other races. For thousands of years soy has been a staple in the Asian diet. So scientists began studying this possible connection and found a link between years of regular soy consumption and decreased rates of breast cancer.

However—and this is where it gets confusing—that hormonal link I mentioned earlier also creates an unknown factor. There's been some talk that women who've been treated for or have a strong family history of breast cancer should avoid soy. More research is being done in this important, yet confusing, area.

For you men, those soy isoflavones can help reduce your risk of getting prostate cancer, and if you already have it, may decrease the chances that it will kill you.

So how much of this stuff do you need? The United States Food and Drug Administration allows a health claim to be on the label of foods containing soy stating that 25 grams of soy protein per day as part of a diet low in saturated fat and cholesterol may help reduce the risk of heart disease. As of now, there are no recommendations for isoflavones; however, it appears that an average intake of about 50 milligrams per day may produce the desired benefits.

Kryptonite _____

If you've been treated for breast cancer or have a first-degree female relative (mother, sister, daughter) with breast cancer, I wouldn't go overboard on soy. That means until more is known, I wouldn't take soy supplements or use a lot of soy powder, both of which contain high amounts of soy isoflavones. However, there's no need to eliminate soy from your diet altogether. An occasional glass of soymilk is okay. A soy burger now and again is fine, too. In fact, because they contain only a small amount of isoflavones, foods such as soy burgers and soy dogs can be eaten more regularly without problems. Remember also, this doesn't mean that you need to stay away from soy sauce or foods listing soybean oil as an ingredient, because these two items don't contain any isoflavones at all.

Now you know what soy can do and how much is needed to obtain the health benefits. The question remaining is, where do you find soy?

First, there are all the different versions of cooked soybeans—whether you eat it or not, you've probably heard of tofu. And increasing in popularity in more recent years are soymilk, soy cheese, and soy yogurt, as well as soy nuts and soy flour. Also popular are all the foods made with soy, like soy burgers and soy dogs.

Protein and Isoflavone Content of Soy Foods

Soy Food	Grams of Protein	Milligrams of Isoflavones
½ Cup of Raw Soybeans	34	140
One Cup of Soy Milk	10	23
Four Ounces of Tofu	18	32
½ Cup of Soy Nuts	30	110

Kryptonite

Foods with soy as an ingredient and soy-based infant formulas are widely consumed by children and are considered completely safe. However, there haven't been studies done on the safety of isolated soy protein (which is created by removing most of the nonprotein components from soybeans, resulting in a product that is almost pure soy protein) or isoflavones supplements in children, so they are not recommended at this time for children's use.

Edamame

Let's start right with the soybean itself. Edamame are fresh green soybeans. They are high in protein and fiber.

Nutrition Information for ½ Cup of Edamame

Calories	100
Total Fat	3 grams
Saturated Fat	0 grams
Trans Fat	0 grams
Cholesterol	0 milligrams
Sodium	260 milligrams
Total Carbohydrate	9 grams
Dietary Fiber	4 grams
Sugars	1 gram
Protein	8 grams
Vitamin A	10% Daily Value
Vitamin C	10% Daily Value
Calcium	6% Daily Value
Iron	10% Daily Value

You can often find them in the freezer section of your grocery store. They are also sometimes available fresh in the salad bar section of larger supermarkets. They've become a popular snack food. To eat them this way, simply boil them in lightly salted water and use your fingers to squeeze the seeds out of the pods and into your mouth. The shelled beans can also be tossed into a salad as you might do with garbanzo beans, or mixed with a pasta dish along with other vegetables.

Soymilk

Probably the most popular soy food on the market today, especially among nonvegetarians, is soymilk.

Nutrition Information for 1 Cup of Soymilk

Calories	130
Total Fat	4.5 grams
Saturated Fat	0.5 grams
Trans Fat	0 grams
Cholesterol	0 milligrams
Sodium	135 milligrams
Total Carbohydrate	12 grams
Dietary Fiber	3 grams
Sugars	1 gram
Protein	11 grams
Vitamin A	30% Daily Value
Calcium	10% Daily Value
Iron	15% Daily Value

It is commonly found in the dairy department of the grocery store right alongside the more traditional cow's milk. Also like traditional milk, you can buy it plain or in flavors like chocolate or vanilla. It also comes in regular or lite, which has less fat. Soymilk is a good source of protein, iron, and several B-vitamins.

Kryptonite

Soymilk is not naturally high in calcium or vitamin D. If you are using it in place of cow's milk, look for a brand that is fortified with these vitamins and minerals.

Because this is not a dairy food, it does not contain *lactose*, and so is an option for those with *lactose intolerance*. It can also be a good substitute for those allergic to cow's milk. You can drink it as is or you can use it as a substitute for cow's milk when baking and cooking. Soymilk is also used to make soy yogurts and cheeses in the same way cow's milk is used to make traditional yogurts and cheeses.

def•i•ni•tion

Lactose is the sugar in milk and milk products. It is broken down in the body by the enzyme lactase.

Lactose intolerance is a condition in which your body doesn't break down lactose due to low levels of lactase. This can result in stomach pain, bloating, gas, and/or diarrhea.

Tofu

Tofu is cooked soybeans puréed into a curd. Tofu is extremely versatile. Because it's very spongelike, it has a tendency to take on whatever flavor you cook it with, whether that be a savory sauce for a dinner or cocoa for a sweet dessert.

Nutrition Information for 3 Ounces of Soft Tofu

Calories	45
Total Fat	2.5 grams
Saturated Fat	0 grams
Trans Fat	0 grams
Cholesterol	0 milligrams
Sodium	0 milligrams
Total Carbohydrate	2 grams
Dietary Fiber	0 grams
Sugars	1 gram
Protein	4 grams
Calcium	2% Daily Value
Iron	4% Daily Value

Typically tofu can be found in the produce department of your grocery store in water-filled containers or vacuum-packed bricks. It is perishable, so be sure to check the expiration date. Once opened, rinse the tofu and recover it with water. Change the water every day and toss out leftovers after 1 week. Tofu freezes well for up to 5 months.

It's available in three main types: firm, soft, and silken. The type you select depends on what you plan to do with it. The firm type holds its shape well and therefore is good in stir-fries or on the grill. The soft version works well when the recipe calls to blend it, such as with soups, sauces, or desserts. The silken works similarly to the soft; it just produces a creamier result.

Not quite sure what to do with it? You can crumble it and use it as a substitute for or mixed with ground beef for tacos, meatloaf, or burgers. Try marinating and grilling cubes of it. Or you could blend it with cocoa or melted chocolate chips and your sweetener of choice for a protein-packed chocolate cream pie.

Miso

Miso is paste made by combining soybeans and a grain like rice with salt and a mold culture.

Nutrition Information for 1 Tablespoon of Miso

Calories	35
Total Fat	1 gram
Saturated Fat	0 grams
Trans Fat	0 grams
Cholesterol	0 milligrams
Sodium	640 milligrams
Total Carbohydrate	5 grams
Dietary Fiber	1 gram
Sugars	1 gram
Protein	2 grams
Iron	2% Daily Value

Miso is used as a condiment to flavor sauces, soups, and marinades or in place of salt or soy sauce. You can find it in natural-food stores, and it will store in the refrigerator for months. You can mix a tablespoon into a cup of hot water to make a vegetarian broth.

Tempeh

Tempeh is cooked, whole soybeans mixed with a grain and cultured with an edible mold.

Nutrition Information for 4 Ounces of Tempeh

Calories	220
Total Fat	12 grams
Saturated Fat	2.5 grams
Trans Fat	N/A
Cholesterol	0 milligrams
Sodium	10 milligrams
Total Carbohydrate	11 grams
Dietary Fiber	N/A
Sugars	N/A
Protein	21 grams
Calcium	15% Daily Value
Iron	15% Daily Value

Tempeh cakes can be found in the freezer section of a natural-food store. It can be kept frozen for months, as well as in the refrigerator for a little over a week.

It can be used in a variety of ways: steam it, marinate it, and then grill it or add cubes of it to chili, spaghetti sauce, soups, or casseroles.

Soy Nuts

Soy nuts are actually roasted soybeans that taste very much like peanuts.

Nutrition Information for 1 Ounce of Roasted, Unsalted Soy Nuts

Calories	130
Total Fat	7 grams
Saturated Fat	1 gram
Trans Fat	N/A
Cholesterol	0 milligrams
Sodium	0 milligrams
Total Carbohydrate	9 grams
Dietary Fiber	1 gram
Sugars	0 grams
Protein	10 grams
Calcium	4% Daily Value
Iron	8% Daily Value

Soy nuts can be found in a natural food store or the health food section of larger supermarkets.

They're available in a variety of flavors including plain, BBQ, spicy, honey roasted, and even chocolate covered. You can eat them as is, sprinkle them on a salad, or use them in place of other nuts when cooking and baking.

Soy nuts are also used to make soy nut butter. This is a great tree-nut-free alternative to peanut butter for anyone with peanut allergies.

Soy Flour

Soy flour is ground roasted soybeans. You may find it in small bags in the baking or natural foods section of your grocery store or sold by bulk in bins in natural food stores.

Nutrition Information for ¼ Cup of Soy Flour

Calories	100
Total Fat	4.5 grams
Saturated Fat	1 gram
Trans Fat	0 grams
Cholesterol	0 milligrams
Sodium	0 milligrams
Total Carbohydrate	9 grams
Dietary Fiber	4 grams
Sugars	0 grams
Protein	7 grams
Calcium	4% Daily Value
Iron	10% Daily Value

To bake with soy flour, you can replace up to a third of the wheat flour called for in your recipe. It contains no gluten—the component that helps bread rise—so using more than 40 percent of the flour needed in a recipe as soy flour isn't recommended. In cooking, soy flour can act as a thickener in gravies and sauces.

Other Soy Foods

Soy, in the form of soy protein concentrate, texturized soy protein, and soy protein isolate, is used as an ingredient in a variety of foods, especially meat alternatives. If you're not a fan of the nutty soybean flavor you may find in foods like soymilk or soy nuts, or if you're not crazy about tofu, don't despair. You can still reap the benefits from soy by including countless other foods made with soy in your diet. These include foods like veggie or soy burgers, soy dogs, and soy bacon and sausage. In fact, you can even find soy-based substitutes for spicy chicken wings and corn dogs.

So whatever your tastes lean to, there's a good chance you can find a way that soy foods can fit into your eating plan.

Yogurt

Yogurt's many health benefits come to us in two ways. First, simply the nature of being a dairy product means that yogurt is full of protein and minerals like calcium. But in addition, the unique health benefits of yogurt come from what makes yogurt yogurt. That is the bacteria that ferments the sweet liquid milk and cream into the slightly tart, creamy concoction we all know.

Nutrition Information for 1 Cup of Plain, Nonfat Yogurt

Calories	100
Total Fat	0 grams
Saturated Fat	0 grams
Trans Fat	0 grams
Cholesterol	5 milligrams
Sodium	135 milligrams
Total Carbohydrate	19 grams
Dietary Fiber	0 grams
Sugars	13 grams
Protein	10 grams
Vitamin A	20% Daily Value
Vitamin C	20% Daily Value
Calcium	30% Daily Value

Yogurt is a great source of protein. One cup or 8 ounces of yogurt contains 10 grams. That's almost twice as much as is in an ounce of beef or one whole egg. One of the bonuses of protein-rich foods is that they are digested slowly. Translation: they help keep you full longer than *carbohydrate*-rich foods like grains and fruits. Keeping hunger pangs at bay is helpful in losing or maintaining weight.

def•i•ni•tion

Carbohydrates are your body's main source of energy. They include sugars, starches, and fiber.

Calcium is another key nutrient found in yogurt. In fact, 1 protein-rich cup has more calcium than an 8-ounce glass of milk. For years we've heard about calcium's role in building strong bones, but it does so much more. In addition to being a key player in osteoporosis prevention, calcium helps regulate your heartbeat. It also has a role in clotting your blood when you get cut. And lately research has shown that calcium is involved with even more important body works.

Blood pressure a bit over the top? Try eating two to three servings of calcium-rich, low-fat foods such as yogurt every day. This along with a diet full of fruits, veggies, and whole grains and keeping your sodium intake to less than 2,500 milligrams per day may be just what you need to get your blood pressure where it should be.

Like to lose a little body fat and get your weight down? Achieving adequate calcium in your diet, primarily from dairy foods, may promote more weight loss compared to folks who don't eat enough of this essential mineral. The bonus is that more of the weight you lose comes from that jelly around

your belly. All you need to do is strive for 1,200–
1,300 milligrams per day. That's a mere three to
four servings of calcium-filled foods such as low-fat
yogurt, milk, and cheese.

Kryptonite

While all yogurt contains sugar due
to the naturally occurring sugar in
milk, some have more added sugar than
others. This can be an issue if you have
diabetes, are watching your weight, or
are just limiting your sugar intake. When
buying yogurt, check the label to compare
brands and styles to find the lowest sugar
content.

And saving the best for last—those bacteria. And
not just any bacteria, we're talking lactic-acid
bacteria, especially lactobacilli and bifidobacteria.
These friendly bacteria are called *probiotics*.

def•i•ni•tion

Probiotics are living microorganisms that
benefit your health beyond the basic strong
body building when they are eaten in
certain amounts.

Before I go any further, you need to know that
to achieve the following benefits, the yogurt you
choose must contain live, active cultures of these

bacteria. It's not as bad as it sounds. Many yogurts do, and you've probably eaten them without knowing it. But you won't find these friendly guys in the yogurt with candy sprinkles to mix in. So if that's the only yogurt in the fridge, it's time for a trip to the market. Look at the ingredient list, where it should say whether or not the product contains live, active cultures.

Probiotics are just full of good deeds for your body, ranging from decreasing diarrhea to possibly preventing stomach cancer and many things in between.

How do they perform all these wondrous feats? Your *gastrointestinal tract* naturally contains hundreds of different types of bacteria. Most are good, but some aren't. When the balance of these bacteria gets disrupted by sickness, stress, or antibiotics, to name a few, the bad bacteria can grow out of control. This overgrowth can lead to a variety of conditions and diseases including diarrhea and yeast infections. Probiotics help keep or restore the healthy balance of bacteria you need.

def•i•ni•tion

The **gastrointestinal tract** can also be called the digestive tract. It's made up of all of the organs involved in digestion including the mouth, stomach, and intestines.

If you've got a weak stomach, you may want to make sure you're seated for the rest of this chapter.

Talking about the gastrointestinal tract isn't often pleasant. Think about it. What goes on down there is digestion. That means stomachaches, gas, and food moving through too quickly or too slowly. See what I mean? Not a lot of fun stuff. So don't say I didn't warn you!

We've all had it at one time or another. You may call it loose bowels, just plain old diarrhea, or worse. Depending on the cause of your problem, eating yogurt on a regular basis may decrease the severity of and possibly even prevent the problem in the first place. This has been seen when the trouble is caused by antibiotic use, rotavirus in young children, and travelers' diarrhea.

Ever have an ulcer? Did you know ulcers are caused by bacteria? The bacteria *Helicobacter pylori* (H. pylori) to be exact. This nasty guy is responsible for some types of gastritis, peptic ulcers, and maybe even stomach cancer.

Probiotics to the rescue again. These powerful, good bacteria may just prevent that bad H. pylori from growing and causing you lots of painful and serious problems. Doing so requires you to eat yogurt on a daily basis.

You've probably been told more than once to take vitamin C to prevent a cold, but how about to take yogurt? Information is just coming out showing that the bacteria in yogurt may give your immune system a boost by increasing your resistance to infections, gastrointestinal problems, and allergies. Stay tuned for more on this emerging area of interest.

Back to those bowels. Since probiotics affect the bacteria of the intestines, they may be helpful if you're suffering from a variety of bowel diseases including *inflammatory bowel syndrome* and *ulcerative colitis*. These diseases often tend to come and go, with periods of remission alternating with periods of symptoms. Regular yogurt consumption may reduce symptoms as well as maintain the remission times.

def•i•ni•tion

Inflammatory bowel syndrome is an intestinal condition characterized by abdominal pain, bloating, and alternating constipation and diarrhea.

Ulcerative colitis is an inflammation of the colon.

And finally, for the millions of Americans suffering from lactose intolerance, probiotics work in a slightly different way. Even though yogurt is a dairy food and therefore contains lactose, it not only may be tolerated but may help those suffering from this uncomfortable and sometimes embarrassing condition.

A diagnosis of lactose intolerance is always followed with an instruction to cut dairy foods out of your diet. Often, however, yogurt is the one food from that group that can be tolerated without symptoms. This is because live yogurt cultures contain the lactase necessary to break down the lactose.

The lactase performs the digestive work the body is unable to, thus eliminating the embarrassing problems that result from undigested sugars.

In addition, probiotics simply improve the way the intestines work. Therefore, eating yogurt on a regular basis may actually decrease your sensitivity to undigested milk sugar.

After all of that, I'd say it'd be tough to find a good reason not to eat yogurt. Whether you're looking for strong bones or a satisfying snack, or you're trying to lose that spare tire around your middle or having some bowel troubles, yogurt can give you the help you need.

The Least You Need to Know

- Even if you're not a tofu fan, there are a variety of foods containing soy you can include in your diet.
- Soy protein and isoflavones are responsible for the many health benefits of soy foods.
- Yogurt can help build strong bones and so much more.
- Good bacteria in yogurt improve or reduce symptoms of an assortment of intestinal ailments.

Chapter 6

Protein Power

In This Chapter

- Fat is good for you?
- Omega-3 isn't a fraternity
- Beans do more than make you toot
- Why you should give turkey a try

What do a fish, a plant, and a bird have in common? The particular ones discussed in this chapter are all excellent sources of protein in your diet. All seafood, as well as beans such as black, kidney, navy, and many more, and poultry provide the body with protein that is essential for building and upholding bodily structures like bone and skin.

Protein also helps to control functions like disease fighting and can be used for energy. In addition, because they are slower to be digested than carbohydrates such as breads, cereals, and grains, protein foods stay in your digestive system longer, helping to keep you feeling more satisfied with your meals and feeling fuller longer.

Super Salmon

Fish, no matter what kind—whitefish, shellfish, coldwater fish, etc.—is an incredibly nutritious food. Not only is it a great source of protein, but that protein is also complete, meaning that it provides you with all the essential amino acids your body needs to develop and work properly. Many types of fish contain virtually no fat or saturated fat. Seafood contains a variety of vitamins and minerals, too.

Salmon in particular is especially healthful even though it contains more fat than most fish. In fact, the fat is what makes salmon so extra-special when it comes to your health.

Nutrition Information for 3 Ounces of Baked or Broiled Salmon

Calories	150
Total Fat	7 grams
Saturated Fat	1 gram
Cholesterol	60 milligrams
Sodium	50 milligrams
Total Carbohydrate	0 grams
Dietary Fiber	0 grams
Sugars	0 grams
Protein	22 grams
Calcium	2% Daily Value
Iron	4% Daily Value

For a long time many people thought that fat in the diet was bad. So, the word got out to cut fat from the diet. The truth is that some fat is necessary. Fat cushions and protects the organs and provides needed vitamins and minerals. In addition, there are different kinds of fat, some of which are good and some of which aren't. You may have heard of harmful saturated and trans fats that increase the risk of heart disease. Then there are the good monounsaturated and polyunsaturated fats.

Turns out that the type of fat you eat affects the production of compounds in your body called eicosanoids, which influence blood pressure, blood clotting, inflammation, and the function of your immune system. An especially healthful group of eicosanoids are produced by *omega-3 fatty acids*. The best source of these fatty acids in your diet is cold-water oily fish. Being a cold-water oily fish, salmon is super-rich in omega-3 fatty acids.

Omega-3 fatty acids don't act alone. They work in conjunction with *omega-6 fatty acids*, sort of. What's truly important to your health is the ratio of omega-3s to omega-6s.

Ideally the ratio of omega-6 to omega-3 should be from 3:1 to 5:1. In the typical Western diet the ratio is somewhere between 10:1 and 30:1. This is unfortunate because excessive amounts of omega-6 acids compared to omega-3 acids may increase the risk of many diseases, including some cancers and cardiovascular disease. Now before you try to eliminate all omega-6 fatty acids from your diet, remember that it's an essential fat. This means your body needs it but can't make it. A better scenario would be to cut down your omega-6 intake while at the same time increasing your omega-3 intake.

def•i•ni•tion

> **Omega-3 fatty acids** are a group of essential polyunsaturated fats found primarily in fish oils, especially salmon, that lower blood cholesterol levels. The three main ones are ALA (alpha-linolenic acid), EPA (eicosapentaenoic acid), and DHA (docosahexaenoic acid).
>
> **Omega-6 fatty acids** are a group of essential fatty acids that compete in the body with omega-3 fatty acids. They are found in cereals, whole-grain breads, most vegetable oils, and baked goods.

One of the big bonuses of boosting your omega-3 intake by eating more salmon is benefiting your heart and cardiovascular system. Omega-3 fatty acids protect against heart attacks in a number of ways. First, they hamper the creation of blood clots; most heart attacks are caused by blood clots blocking the blood vessels going to the heart. In addition, they may slow the growth of plaque that builds up and narrows the heart's arteries. They also may help prevent heartbeat abnormalities, which protects against sudden cardiac death—a major cause of heart-disease death. Omega-3 fatty acids also help to lower blood cholesterol levels, including total cholesterol, LDL, and triglycerides. High levels of these fats in your blood increase your risk of having a heart attack.

Through another avenue toward a healthy cardio-vascular system, omega-3s help battle hypertension. Researchers studying blood pressure found that both eating less fat and eating more fish lowered participants' blood pressure. When both dietary changes were combined, blood pressure decreased even more than with each change individually.

The omega-6 to omega-3 ratio also plays a part in cancer protection. Omega-6 fatty acids are known to enhance the development, growth, and spread of cancerous tumors. However, decreasing your intake of omega-6s along with increasing your intake of omega-3s has been shown to be related to lower incidences of breast cancer. A similar relationship is seen with prostate cancer. One large study showed that non-fish-eating men developed prostate cancer two to three times more than men who ate fish regularly. It appears that omega-3 fatty acids reduce the activity of an enzyme called COX-2. This enzyme works with omega-6 fatty acids to promote the development of new blood vessels needed for tumor growth. By reducing the COX-2 activity, omega-3s assist in slowing or stopping the new blood vessel growth.

If you suffer from rheumatoid arthritis (RA), here's some news for you. Adequate intake of omega-3 fatty acids may reduce the pain from RA in just a few months—and, if eaten regularly, may also improve grip strength and possibly result in the need for less medication. For those of you without RA, eating salmon can lower your risk of developing it. But you should know that for some reason this effect was seen only when the fish was broiled or baked.

Omega-3s are also involved in mental health. Low levels of these fatty acids in the diet are linked to increased rates of depression. And in those over the age of 75, higher levels of DHA (docosahexaenoic acid) in the blood can significantly reduce the risk of dementia, including Alzheimer's, compared to those with low levels. A great way to boost blood levels of DHA is eating fatty fish, like salmon, regularly.

Omega-3 fatty acids, specifically DHA, are even helpful for those of us not yet there. DHA helps the brain develop; the most rapid time for this work is 3 months before and 3 months after birth. The benefits continue up until the age of 2, but more slowly. So if you're pregnant or breastfeeding, make sure salmon is a regular part of your weekly menu.

So how much salmon should you be eating? The American Heart Association recommends including fish, especially fatty fish, in your diet at least twice a week. While this is for heart health, the recommendation seems to be consistent to achieve all the benefits I've discussed. Eating fish this often will provide sufficient amounts of omega-3 fatty acids.

Both wild and farmed salmon provide the same benefits nutritionally speaking. They are both great sources of protein and omega-3 fatty acids. However, there are important differences you should know. Wild salmon can be caught only between May and September and tends to be expensive, about $15 per pound. To increase availability and cut costs, farmed salmon entered the picture. Farmed salmon is available year-round at a price closer to $6 per pound. Sounds good, right? Well, it can be, but it does have a downside.

In addition to polluting the shoreline and reducing the amount of fish available for humans to eat, farmed salmon are contaminated with industrial chemicals and could increase your risk of cancer. Scientists of all kinds have looked into this issue and developed guidelines. When selecting your salmon, choose fish raised in Chile and Washington State. Avoid fish from Scotland and the Faroe Islands. Also, when cooking, score the flesh and grill or broil, so the juices drip off, until an internal temperature of 175° Fahrenheit is reached, and remove the skin before eating. These simple steps could remove half of the harmful contaminants. The recommendations are to eat no more than 6 ounces of cooked farmed salmon per month. However, following the steps above enables you to eat up to 12 ounces per month.

Most importantly, don't give up eating salmon. Farmed salmon decreases your risk of dying from a heart attack much more than it increases your risk of cancer.

Beans, Beans the Magical Fruit

The schoolyard rhyme has really given beans a bad name. Sure, they may make you toot, but it's because of one of the very properties that make them so good for you—the fiber.

Nutrition Information for ½ Cup of Cooked Black Beans

Calories	110
Total Fat	0 grams
Saturated Fat	0 grams
Trans Fat	0 grams
Cholesterol	0 milligrams
Sodium	0 milligrams
Total Carbohydrate	20 grams
Dietary Fiber	7 grams
Sugars	1 gram
Protein	8 grams
Calcium	2% Daily Value
Iron	10% Daily Value

Beans are full of a variety of nutrients. These include protein, B vitamins like folate, minerals like iron, and soluble and insoluble fiber. It's also important to note what they don't contain that helps make them so healthy. They contain no sodium, cholesterol, or saturated fat, and they are very low in calories.

Kryptonite

The nutrition information for beans is based on beans cooked from dry, which, as the chart shows, contain no sodium. Canned beans, however, do contain a good deal of sodium, but are much more convenient. To drastically reduce the sodium in canned beans, simply rinse them well before using.

Beans are one example of what are known as low-GI foods. GI stands for glycemic index and it's a measure of how foods affect your blood sugar levels and your body's insulin response after eating. When you eat, food is turned into sugar, or glucose, to be used by your body. In response, your body releases the hormone insulin to help move the glucose from the blood to the tissues that need it. Some foods, such as sugar and white bread, which are known as high-GI foods, make your blood sugar rise very quickly, causing insulin levels to rise quickly as well. The insulin then causes the blood sugar levels to drop rapidly. Frequent fluctuations of these two substances are associated with several negative consequences such as increased hunger, which could lead to weight gain from eating more frequently, and a decreased sensitivity to insulin, which could lead to diabetes.

Low-GI foods such as beans offer many health benefits. They keep you full longer after eating, which could help with weight loss and maintenance. They increase the body's sensitivity to insulin, helping it respond more efficiently. Low-GI foods also help reduce your risk of heart disease and can lower your cholesterol levels.

Beans also contain substances called oligosaccharides, which are *prebiotics*. These prebiotics improve the health of your digestive tract, specifically your colon.

def•i•ni•tion

> **Prebiotics** are undigestible carbohydrates in foods that encourage the growth of good bacteria in the intestines.

Increased amounts of good bacteria in your intestines are associated with lower cholesterol levels, enhanced immune function, and improved mineral absorption. In addition, these beneficial bacteria increase the colon's acidity, making it tough for disease-causing organisms like viruses and bad bacteria to survive.

The fact that beans contain no sodium or saturated fat makes them a perfect heart-healthy food, but they go beyond not increasing your risk of heart disease. Eating beans can actually decrease your risk. Beans contain *plant sterols*, which lower cholesterol levels. The combination of a diet including plant sterols and regular exercise has been shown to lower both total and LDL cholesterol as well as triglyceride levels. These two factors also increase HDL cholesterol levels.

def•i•ni•tion

Plant sterols are plant-based substances that compete with cholesterol for absorption by the intestines. By doing so, they help lower cholesterol levels.

The soluble fiber found in beans also helps lower cholesterol levels. A decrease of just 1 percent in total cholesterol is linked to about a 2–4 percent drop in risk of developing heart disease. In other words, if your cholesterol is 225mg/dL and you drop it to the recommended 200, that's about a 9 percent reduction and would correlate to at least an 18 percent reduced risk of developing heart disease.

Beans are a good source of the vitamin folate, which also plays a role in preventing heart disease. High levels of an amino acid called homocysteine in your blood are a risk factor for developing cardiovascular disease. Folate works to lower that risk by helping to lower homocysteine levels. Just a half cup of beans provides about one quarter of your daily folate needs.

Speaking of folate and homocysteine—low levels of folate and high levels of homocysteine may make the brain cells more susceptible to damage.

Increasing folate in the diet by eating more foods like beans and thus lowering homocysteine levels can help prevent this damage and could significantly lower your risk of developing Alzheimer's disease.

Beans are active in cancer prevention, too. A recent study found that women who ate beans at least twice a week had a lower risk of breast cancer. This study was done after noticing that countries where bean consumption was the highest had the lowest number of deaths from breast, prostate, and colon cancer. In addition, obesity, or excess body fat, increases your risk of several types of cancer. Being a low-GI food and helping with weight maintenance is a second way that beans can help reduce your risk of cancer.

Super Knowledge

We can't forget the reason many folks shy away from beans—the gas. There is a way to enjoy beans and obtain their many health benefits without having to leave the room every few minutes. Beano to the rescue. Beano is an enzyme that helps digest the sugars in beans and other foods to make them less gassy. It's not a drug, and you can find it easily in supermarkets and drugstores. All you do is take it with your meal, and problem solved.

Terrific Turkey

Again I find myself thinking of the Thanksgiving table with that deep-brown roasted turkey sitting in the middle surrounded by sweet potatoes and pumpkin dishes and more.

Nutrition Information for 3 Ounces of Skinless Roasted Turkey Breast

Calories	110
Total Fat	0.5 grams
Saturated Fat	0 grams
Cholesterol	70 milligrams
Sodium	45 milligrams
Total Carbohydrate	0 grams
Dietary Fiber	0 grams
Sugars	0 grams
Protein	26 grams
Calcium	2% Daily Value
Iron	8% Daily Value

It seems we eat well at least one day of the year, though there is a tendency to overdo it. Now it's my job to convince you to eat all of these foods more often to reap their many benefits. And turkey is definitely one of them—turkey breast without the skin, to be exact.

Skinless turkey breast is second only to seafood when it comes to lean animal protein sources. And that's a close second. It contains very little fat and virtually none of the heart-clogging saturated fat found in most animal products. Turkey breast is also very low in sodium. These virtues by themselves are enough to qualify skinless turkey breast as healthy for your heart. Organizations like the American Heart Association recommend eating a diet low in fat, saturated fat, and sodium for optimum heart health, so you can see why they'd love skinless turkey breasts.

But that's not all. Turkey is stuffed with a variety of vitamins, minerals, and other nutrients you can be thankful for.

Turkey is a rich source of niacin, which is in what is called the B-complex vitamin family. The B-vitamins—riboflavin and thiamin are two more—are involved in energy production in your body. Niacin is necessary to help convert protein, fat, and carbohydrates from the foods you eat into a form of energy that your body can use. Niacin is also used to create a form of energy that is stored in your muscles and liver to be used later when needed. In addition, niacin is essential for synthesis of various hormones, including insulin, and is part of glucose tolerance factor, which is a compound that enhances the body's response to insulin.

Niacin has been looked at with regard to cognitive decline issues such as Alzheimer's disease. A study found that those regularly eating about 50 percent more than the RDA were significantly less likely to develop Alzheimer's disease than those eating less than the RDA. One 4-ounce serving of roasted turkey provides about half of the RDA for niacin.

Turkey is also an excellent source of *tryptophan*. Yes, this is that substance in turkey that everyone blames for putting them to sleep after Thanksgiving dinner. While tryptophan is involved in sleep regulation, the famous turkey-day snooze is more likely due to eating a huge meal and then sitting around on the couch watching the parade or football. But I digress. Tryptophan is an essential amino acid, meaning that your body needs it to make the proteins it needs. It's well known for helping in the production of nervous-system messengers involved in relaxation, restfulness, and sleep. Tryptophan is converted to *serotonin* in the body, which explains why it helps with relaxation.

def•i•ni•tion

Tryptophan is one of the 10 essential amino acids the body uses for protein synthesis.

Serotonin is a neurotransmitter involved in the regulation of appetite, sleep, and mood.

While most of the tryptophan we eat gets turned into serotonin, a very small amount is converted into niacin. When someone has a very low intake of niacin, this conversion occurs to help prevent symptoms of niacin deficiency. Because turkey is such a great source of niacin as well as tryptophan, it works double duty in promoting the health benefits niacin offers.

While there is no official RDA for tryptophan, scientists at the National Academy of Sciences, where the RDAs are developed, have come up with an unofficial recommendation. Based on protein requirements, they've determined that adult men should get 392 milligrams and adult women need 322 milligrams. Just one 4-ounce serving of roasted turkey contains 350 milligrams.

Turkey is also a good source of zinc. Zinc is a mineral your body needs every day, but only in very small amounts. Zinc is involved in a number of processes in your body. These include regulating gene activity. Without enough zinc, the cells in your body may not be able to know what your genes are directing them to do.

Zinc is also involved in maintaining metabolism and blood sugar levels. Without enough zinc, it becomes hard to stabilize blood sugar levels. This is especially dangerous for people with diabetes, who must work hard to keep their blood sugar around a certain level. In addition, inadequate zinc can cause your metabolic rate to drop. The metabolic rate is the rate at which your body uses up the calories from the foods you eat. A slower rate means fewer calories are needed to maintain body weight, and it may make gaining weight easier.

Zinc has a role in the functioning of your senses, too. Zinc must be present for you to smell and taste properly. And zinc is needed to enable your immune system to function at its best.

All along I've been talking about skinless turkey breast, but when you go to the grocery store, you should know there are several options available to achieve the benefits I've shared. Turkey tenderloins, cutlets, and medallions all come from the turkey breast. Just be sure to remove the skin if it isn't already gone. Broiling, baking, or grilling these turkey cuts as well as breasts are ideal ways to cook them while maintaining their nutritional quality.

The Least You Need to Know

- Healthy fats protect you from diseases like cancer and heart disease.

- Farmed and wild salmon are both good for you, but farmed salmon may be contaminated with industrial chemicals that could increase your risk of cancer. When cooking, score the flesh and grill or broil, so the juices drip off, until an internal temperature of 175° Fahrenheit is reached, and remove the skin before eating.

- Beans and other low-GI foods offer many benefits including assistance with controlling your weight.

- Skinless turkey breasts are extremely low in fat but high in nutrition.

Chapter 7

Fields of Dreams

In This Chapter

- Oatmeal, a great start to your day
- Adding oats and flax to your diet can boost flavor and fiber
- Get *flax*-ible
- What to do with flaxseeds

I've told you about fruits and vegetables. We've covered protein and dairy. There's even been talk of some drinks. So what's left? Those glorious grains! We can't forget all the good they do for us.

Oh, Those Oats

What is there not to like about oats? They're tasty, easy to prepare, and cheap. And if those aren't enough, wait until you find out all the good work they do for you.

Nutrition Information for 1 Cup of Cooked Oatmeal

Calories	130
Total Fat	2 grams
Saturated Fat	0 grams
Cholesterol	0 milligrams
Sodium	105 milligrams
Total Carbohydrate	22 grams
Dietary Fiber	4 grams
Sugars	0 grams
Protein	5 grams
Vitamin A	25% Daily Value
Calcium	15% Daily Value
Iron	60% Daily Value

Oats are considered whole grains. While refined grains like white rice and white flour are made by removing the germ and the bran of the grain, whole grains include these two parts. And it's these two components that contain much of the fiber, vitamins, minerals, phytochemicals, and other important nutrients found in grains.

Oats historically have been known to protect against heart disease. In fact, those who eat two and a half to three servings of whole grains per day cut their risk of coronary heart disease by one quarter compared to those who don't eat them.

In addition, in the many indirect ways that oats achieve this goal, they are also beneficial for other diseases.

Super Knowledge

The 2005 Dietary Guidelines for Americans recommends eating at least three servings of whole grains per day to lower your risk of many chronic diseases. Whole grains include oatmeal, brown rice, popcorn, dark breads, and whole-grain breakfast cereals. One serving is considered 1 half cup of cooked grain, 1 ounce of cold cereal, 1 slice of bread, and 2 cups of popcorn.

The fiber in oats is mainly responsible for their nutritional benefits. The first part of improving your heart-disease risk involves lowering cholesterol. Oats are one of the richest sources of a specific type of soluble fiber called beta-glucan.

Beta-glucan is an insoluble fiber that can hold water and forms a thick, gel-like liquid. This gel binds with bile acids and increases their excretion. The body responds by using cholesterol to make more bile acids, therefore lowering cholesterol levels in the blood. In addition, soluble fiber slows the rate at which food goes through your digestive tract. This in turn results in less insulin circulating, which slows the formation of cholesterol. Soluble fiber may also decrease the amount of cholesterol that is absorbed by the intestines.

Studies have shown oats improving cholesterol levels by as much as 23 percent.

And while many studies investigating cholesterol show results primarily in people with high cholesterol levels, oats appear to lower cholesterol in people with normal cholesterol levels, too. Most studies involve improvements in total and LDL cholesterol, but several have also involved HDL cholesterol. Oats have been shown to increase this good cholesterol.

Oats have proven to be so helpful to heart health that in 1997 the U.S. Food and Drug Administration recognized them for it. The FDA allowed the first-ever food-specific health claim, stating that the soluble fiber in oat foods may lower the risk of heart disease in a low-saturated fat and low-cholesterol diet. The recommended goal is 3 grams of oat beta-glucan per day to lower total cholesterol by an average of 6 mg/dL. Remember, just a 1 percent drop in cholesterol corresponds to a 2–4 percent drop in heart disease risk. Each half cup of cooked oats, or quarter cup of uncooked oats (could be used to sprinkle on yogurt, etc.), provides 1 gram of beta-glucan.

Having diabetes increases your risk of developing heart disease. Oats decrease the risk of developing diabetes and also improve blood sugar control in those who already have the disease. Doing so offers another way in which oats lower your risk of heart disease.

The cholesterol-lowering gel solution that beta-glucan fiber forms also works in diabetes. This gel mixture slows the speed at which nutrients are absorbed, which means blood sugar levels and therefore insulin levels remain more consistent versus rising rapidly.

Oats are also beneficial in helping lower blood pressure. By doing so, they lower your risk of developing heart disease, for which high blood pressure is a risk factor.

Kryptonite

High blood pressure is defined as your systolic pressure (the top number) being greater than 140 mm Hg, or your diastolic pressure (the bottom number) being greater than 90 mm Hg. High blood pressure, or hypertension, increases your risk of heart disease by putting extra stress on your arteries. This stress makes the lining of your arteries more susceptible to damage done by LDL, thus increasing your risk of coronary artery disease.

Once again, the fiber is doing most of the work. Studies have demonstrated that people who eat 6 to 10 grams of fiber each day have slightly lower blood pressures than those who eat only 2 to 4 grams. And those eating the recommended daily amount of fiber had a greater than 50 percent reduced risk of developing high blood pressure than those who ate less than half that amount. These results were seen specifically from soluble fiber, the kind oats are high in. People eating more fiber from wheat, the insoluble kind, did not obtain the same results. Certainly wheat fiber is healthy for other reasons, but in this particular instance it's clearly the soluble oat fiber responsible for the healthy improvements.

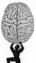 **Super Knowledge**

The U.S. Dietary guidelines recommend that adults over the age of 18 eat 25 to 30 grams of fiber per day. For kids age 2 and above, fiber recommendations are based on age. The American Academy of Pediatrics recommends "5 plus their age" to determine daily fiber needs. For example, a 3-year-old would need 8 grams while a 14-year-old would need 19 grams.

One final way oats indirectly lower your risk of cardiovascular disease is helping control obesity. Obesity is certainly an unhealthy condition on its own, but it is also a risk factor for developing heart disease. In addition, it worsens other heart disease risk factors such as high cholesterol, high blood pressure, and high blood sugar.

One way in which obesity is defined is by your BMI, or body mass index. BMI measures body fatness, which is a more accurate predictor of disease risk than just weight. A BMI between 18.5 and 24.9 is considered normal. Twenty-five to 29.9 is over-weight. Thirty to 39.9 is obese, and a BMI of greater than 40 is morbid or extreme obesity.

Super Knowledge

There are many online calculators to help you determine your BMI—simply use your favorite search engine. To calculate it manually yourself, multiply your height in inches by itself and divide that number into your weight in pounds. Multiply the result by 703. The answer is your BMI.

Several studies on obesity and fiber have produced similar results. One showed that eating 5 to 30 grams per day of both soluble and insoluble fiber can decrease the amount of food you eat as well as your hunger, and produce long-lasting weight loss. In addition, people meeting their fiber needs weigh less than those eating only half that amount. And when it comes to oats, people who included oats as a part of their daily diet lost more weight compared to those who didn't eat oats regularly.

Oats are available in many different forms. There are regular or old-fashioned oats, quick-cooking oats, and instant oatmeal. No matter which type you choose, they all provide the same benefits to your health. However, be aware that the flavored instant oatmeal packets contain more sodium and sugar than plain oatmeal.

Fun with Flax

Remember those omega-3 fats from Chapter 6? Well, they're back in just a slightly different form.

Nutrition Information for 1 Tablespoon of Ground Flaxseeds

Calories	45
Total Fat	3.5 grams
Saturated Fat	0 grams
Trans Fat	0 grams
Cholesterol	0 milligrams
Sodium	0 milligrams
Total Carbohydrate	2 grams
Dietary Fiber	2 grams
Sugars	0 grams
Protein	1 gram
Calcium	2% Daily Value
Iron	2% Daily Value
Omega-3 Fat	1.85 grams
Omega-6 Fat	0.48 grams

Recall the three main types of omega-3s—EPA, DHA, and ALA. Fatty fish like salmon are rich sources of the first two, but for the last one you'd better get yourself some flax. In fact, flaxseeds and flax oil are the richest source of ALA in the American diet. ALA is an essential fat, which means it is "essential" for your body to function properly. EPA and DHA, on the other hand, while extremely beneficial to your health, are not essential. That's because your body makes them from, of all things, ALA.

In addition to omega-3 fatty acids, flax contains high amounts of fiber and substances called *lignans*.

def•i•ni•tion

Lignans are plant compounds that work as both phytoestrogens (plant substances that weakly replicate the action of the hormone estrogen) and antioxidants. These attributes are responsible for many health benefits.

These three components—omega-3s, fiber, and lignans—are responsible for the variety of benefits that flaxseeds offer. Lignans appear to offer protection from breast cancer. Good bacteria in the digestive tract turns plant lignans into substances called enterolactone and enterodiol. These are hormone-like compounds that protect against breast cancer. A recent study showed that high levels of enterolactone in a woman's blood are associated with a substantial decrease in the risk of developing breast cancer in premenopausal women.

The hormone activity that lignans exert can help women achieve hormonal balance by encouraging normal ovulation and lengthening the second half of the menstrual cycle. Normal ovulation means an enhanced likelihood of becoming pregnant for women trying to conceive. The second half of a woman's cycle is the progesterone-heavy half. During peri-menopause, levels of this hormone drop while estrogen levels vary, causing symptoms like headaches, fluid retention, mood swings, weight gain, and other undesirable symptoms associated with peri-menopause. By extending the length of the cycle's second half, lignans found in flax help maintain progesterone levels and thus an even hormonal balance, helping reduce or prevent the above problems.

Kryptonite

The hormonal effect that lignans may have on a developing fetus has not yet been studied adequately. For this reason I'd recommend against using flax products while pregnant or breastfeeding until more information is available.

On a similar note, there's no research on the effect lignans may have on hormone levels during growth and development. So parents are advised to not feed flax to infants and young children regularly. Eating an occasional flax product should be fine, but it shouldn't be included in their diets on a daily basis until more is known.

Back to those fatty acids. ALA provides various benefits for your health. It helps your eyes in two separate ways. First, it may help prevent macular degeneration and, therefore, the blindness to which it can lead. A high intake of omega-6 fatty acid appears to increase the likelihood of developing this disease; however, lower intakes of omega-6 combined with high intakes of omega-3 decreases your chances. In addition, a balanced ratio of omega-3 and omega-6 fatty acids offers a lower risk of developing a painful condition called dry eye syndrome (DES). DES afflicts mostly women and occurs when the quality and quantity of moisturizing tears is reduced, leading to irritation, dryness, a gritty feeling, and, if untreated, possibly vision loss. A recent study showed that a ratio of omega-6 to omega-3 of greater than 15:1, which is similar to the typical American diet, increases the risk of developing DES. Typical treatment is the frequent use of artificial tears. But it appears that a lower ratio, in other words, more omega-3s and less omega-6s, resulted in a substantially reduced risk. It helps by ensuring an adequate amount and consistency of oil to coat the eye's surface, which prevents the tear layer covering the eye from evaporating.

Flax decreases the amount of compounds called cell adhesion molecules in the blood. These molecules increase the creation of plaques, which stick to artery walls blocking blood flow. Plaques can also burst, causing clots that can lead to heart attacks and strokes. By lowering levels of these molecules, flax can prevent or slow heart disease progression.

Flax has also been shown to lower cholesterol levels. In fact, a study in which ground flaxseed was compared to a frequently used type of cholesterol-lowering medicine showed similar reductions in total cholesterol, LDL cholesterol, and triglycerides from both treatments.

Omega-3 fats also help promote flexible cell membranes. Cell membrane flexibility allows for efficient flow of material in and out of cells. This is especially important if you have diabetes, because the more flexible the cell membranes, the more responsive they are to insulin and allowing glucose to go where it needs to go. Alternatively, diets high in *saturated fat* and *trans fats* lead to stiff cell membranes, thus decreased sensitivity to insulin and potentially higher blood glucose levels.

def•i•ni•tion

Trans fat is a type of fatty acid created when liquid fats, or oils, are hydrogenated to make them solid. This is done to make the fat more stable and to increase its shelf life. Trans fats are far worse than the dreaded saturated fat because trans fats raise LDL, or bad cholesterol. Trans fats are found in solid shortening, solid or stick margarines, crackers, baked goods, and other snack foods.

Saturated fat is a fat that is solid at room temperature, like butter and meat fat. It raises cholesterol levels, as opposed to unsaturated fat, which is liquid at room temperature (think olive or canola oil) and tends to lower cholesterol levels.

One final task of omega-3 fats involves inflammation, which plays a role in a number of diseases. ALA works with the lignans in flax to help decrease inflammation by producing anti-inflammatory molecules called prostaglandins. Fatty acids made by the omega-3s can help decrease inflammation in diseases like asthma, arthritis, and migraine headaches.

A protein called C-reactive protein, or CRP, increases with inflammation. High levels of this protein are associated with heart disease and insulin resistance—a risk factor for Type 2 diabetes and high blood pressure. ALA and lignans work to decrease the body's reaction that leads to the release of CRP. By doing so, they lower your risk of these conditions.

Kryptonite

If you have diverticulitis, a condition where pockets form and become irritated in the intestine, ground flaxseeds may bother you. If this happens, the oil is probably the best choice for you.

Flax can be purchased as whole seeds, ground seeds, or as oil. Ground seeds are the preferred form because it allows for maximum nutrient absorption. Whole seeds pass through the digestive system undigested, and oil doesn't contain the fiber that the seeds do. Seeds are available in two colors— reddish brown or golden brown—but nutritionally speaking, they are the same. The recommended daily amount of flaxseed is about 1–2 tablespoons of ground seeds per day, or 1 teaspoon of flax oil.

Flax can be incorporated into your diet in a variety of ways. Ground seeds can be sprinkled on cereals or yogurt. They can be added to pancake or muffin mixes or other baked goods. You can mix them into meatballs or meatloaf, or coat chicken or fish with them before baking. Flax oil can be mixed with vinegar and used as a salad dressing.

The Least You Need to Know

- Soluble fiber from foods like oats can lower your risk of heart disease.

- Your BMI is an important number to keep track of. To determine yours, multiply your height in inches by itself and divide that number into your weight in pounds. Multiply the result by 703.

- Eating less omega-6 fatty acid foods while eating more omega-3 fatty acid foods, like flax and fish, can have a tremendous impact on your health.

- To maximize nutrient quality, grind your own flaxseeds.

Sometimes You Feel Like a Nut

In This Chapter

- Do you know what body part the inside of a walnut resembles?
- Nuts: they won't necessarily make you gain weight
- Peanut butter sandwiches aren't just for kids
- Ways to add nuts to your usual diet

"I can't eat nuts; they're too fattening." A response somewhere along those lines is usually what I get after encouraging people to eat nuts for various health reasons. True, nuts contain fat and can be high in calories, but you'll soon learn why the calories may not be an issue and the fat is good.

The Wonder of Walnuts

Bet you didn't know that when a walnut in its shell is cracked open from top to bottom, it looks like a heart. Maybe that's nature's little way of trying to tell us something.

Nutrition Information for 1 Ounce of Walnuts (About 8–10 Nuts)

Calories	190
Total Fat	18 grams
Saturated Fat	1.5 grams
Trans Fat	0 grams
Cholesterol	0 milligrams
Sodium	0 milligrams
Total Carbohydrate	4 grams
Dietary Fiber	2 grams
Sugars	1 gram
Protein	4 grams
Calcium	2% Daily Value
Iron	4% Daily Value
Omega-3 Fat	2.57 grams
Omega-6 Fat	10.8 grams

Walnuts are rich in many nutrients, including melatonin. Remember that sleep hormone I mentioned way back when I told you about cherries? Melatonin is involved in the regulation of sleep and wake cycles and it also has antioxidant powers. Eating walnuts triples the amount of melatonin circulating in the blood; therefore it can help improve sleep, especially if you have jet lag or happen to work the night shift. In addition, as an antioxidant, melatonin protects your body from the damage of free radicals. By doing so, eating walnuts may offer protection against cancer and delay or reduce aging diseases as well as neurodegenerative diseases like Alzheimer's and Parkinson's.

Walnuts also offer benefits to people with diabetes. If you remember, while diabetes is a disease on its own, having it also makes you more susceptible to heart disease. Because of their high polyunsaturated fat content, including walnuts in your diet makes it very easy, if you have diabetes, to achieve your polyunsaturated-fat intake goals. Doing so can improve LDL levels as well as improve the ratio of HDL levels to total cholesterol. When eaten as part of a moderate fat diet, these resulting improvements are even greater than the changes caused by a low-fat diet alone. Walnuts also appear to improve insulin resistance, therefore allowing sugar in the blood to go into the cells that need it.

Walnuts are another great source of the omega-3 fatty acid ALA. This is one of the reasons walnuts are so good for your heart. Regularly including walnuts in your diet can benefit your heart health in many ways. Eating walnuts can lower levels of both C-reactive protein and plaque adhesion molecules. If you recall, these are two factors that signify artery inflammation and therefore are a heart disease risk. By lowering these levels you can lower your risk of heart disease. And even if you don't have diabetes, walnuts can improve your blood cholesterol profile. They can significantly decrease the LDL cholesterol, the bad stuff, and total cholesterol levels; and may increase or at least maintain HDL cholesterol, the good stuff.

Omega-3s help your heart health in other ways, too. They can help make blood platelets less likely to stick together and form clots and block arteries. They can help maintain the regularity of your heartbeat and prevent cardiac arrest, which, unless treated quickly, is fatal.

Super Knowledge

Because of their high fat content, walnuts can easily spoil or go rancid. To lengthen their shelf life, store shelled nuts in an airtight container in the fridge for up to 6 months or the freezer for up to a year. For walnuts in the shell, store in a cool, dark, dry place for up to 6 months.

Walnuts may also improve the health of the cells lining your arteries. They contain an essential amino acid called l-arginine. The body turns l-arginine into nitric acid. Remember, this is the substance that keeps blood vessel linings smooth and able to relax. This allows blood vessels to withstand increased blood flow when they need to. This is beneficial with high blood pressure, diabetes, and other heart problems.

You would think that because walnuts are so high in calories and fat they would cause you to gain weight if you began eating them. But that's not necessarily true. In all of the studies showing how beneficial walnuts are, participants who ate walnuts did not gain any significant amount of weight. In fact, people said they felt less hungry and it was easier to stick to a diet when walnuts were included. This is most likely due to the fat and protein in walnuts. Like protein, fat takes longer to digest than carbohydrates. This results in feelings of full-ness lasting longer and delayed hunger, thus less munching.

Kryptonite

It's true that nuts, including walnuts, contain a significant amount of fat and calories, but this doesn't automatically mean you'll need to go up a clothing size if you start eating them. You can achieve all the benefits I've told you about from just eating one serving of nuts a day. In fact, some studies show results from just one serving per week. A serving of most nuts is an ounce or about a quarter cup. So go ahead and enjoy nuts, just keep an eye on your portions.

Walnuts are good brain food, too. The membranes of your body's cells are mostly made up of fat. This includes your brain cells. These membranes con-trol what goes into and out of the cell. The more omega-3 fats in your diet, the better your brain cells work. Because omega-3 fats are very flexible, they not only encourage nutrients into brain cells but they help flush waste out of them more easily. And a well-nourished cell that's not bogged down with waste works better. This is especially important when we're talking about your brain.

Walnuts are also a rich source of a specific form of vitamin E called gamma-tocopherol. This form of the vitamin may stop the growth of prostate and lung cancer cells.

Can't think of what to do with walnuts? Of course you could just eat them as is, but there are so many other ways to get them into your diet. Try sprinkling them on your breakfast cereal or your salad at lunch. You could also chop them finely and use them to coat fish before baking, or sprinkle into sautéed vegetables for a crunchy dinner. And don't forget you can add them to muffins or quick breads like banana bread, zucchini muffins, or apple pancakes.

The Power of Peanuts

Who would have thought that the favorite sandwich filling of children across the country could actually be good for us?

Nutrition Information for 1 Ounce of Peanuts, Unsalted (About 28 Nuts)

Calories	170
Total Fat	14 grams

Saturated Fat	2 grams
Trans Fat	0 grams
Cholesterol	0 milligrams
Sodium	0 milligrams
Total Carbohydrate	6 grams
Dietary Fiber	2 grams
Sugars	1 gram
Protein	7 grams
Calcium	2% Daily Value
Iron	4% Daily Value

Many adults have let the ever-popular peanut butter sandwich fade out of their lives along with their jump ropes and skateboards, but you may want to take a step back in time once you learn about all the benefits of peanut butter. Heck, you may also want to dust off those jump ropes and skateboards while you're at it—they're great ways to exercise and to have fun at the same time!

Peanuts really pack a nutritional punch. They are good sources of fiber, vitamin E, protein, folate, and more nutrients that provide tremendous health benefits.

I've talked about fiber a good deal so far. Fiber helps lower your risk of heart disease and diabetes. One of the ways it does this is by lowering total and LDL cholesterol levels. Another way is by helping to maintain healthy blood sugar levels. Fiber also aids your digestive system by helping prevent constipation. Fiber also helps fill you up and keep you full, so it's helpful when trying to lose or maintain weight. Unfortunately, the majority of Americans don't take in nearly enough fiber. In fact, many of us only get about half of the recommended daily amount of 30 grams per day. Just one serving of peanuts, which is 1 ounce or 2 tablespoons of peanut butter, has the same amount of fiber as one slice of whole-wheat bread. Make yourself a sandwich and there's about one fifth of your fiber needs for the day.

Nutrition Information for 2 Tablespoons of Peanut Butter

Calories	190
Total Fat	16 grams
Saturated Fat	3 grams
Trans Fat	0 grams
Cholesterol	0 milligrams
Sodium	150 milligrams
Total Carbohydrate	7 grams
Dietary Fiber	2 grams
Sugars	3 grams
Protein	8 grams
Iron	4% Daily Value

Vitamin E is fat-soluble, meaning that it needs fat to be properly absorbed by the body. Because peanuts contain a good amount of healthy fat, obtaining your vitamin E from peanuts or peanut butter means you're not only getting the vitamin but you're also maximizing your absorption of it. It's estimated that up to three quarters of Americans don't eat enough vitamin E to meet their body's needs. That's a shame, because in addition to being an essential vitamin, E is also a powerful antioxidant. Studies show that compared to people who eat very little vitamin E, those who ate adequate amounts have a significantly lower risk of developing Alzheimer's disease. Vitamin E also enhances the work of the immune system. The good news is that just one serving of peanuts provides about 15–20 percent of your vitamin E needs.

Peanuts contain the most protein of all the nuts. Protein is a key player in building and maintaining body structure. It's also beneficial when trying to lose weight because it's more satiating than carbohydrates. Translation: it keeps you feeling full longer.

The vitamin folate helps lower the levels of the amino acid homocysteine in the blood. High levels of this amino acid can damage arteries and lead to heart disease. Lowering homocysteine levels can decrease the risk of heart disease. Folate is also an especially important nutrient for pregnant women and those of child-bearing age. Adequate folate intake, especially in the first several weeks of pregnancy and even before conception, can help prevent neural tube birth defects such as spina bifida.

Peanuts are also a good source of resveratrol. If you remember, this is a powerful phytochemical found in high amounts in red wine. Believe it or not, peanuts contain it, too. Resveratrol can improve the flow of blood to the brain. By doing so, it can lower your risk of having a stroke. It also helps lower your risk of heart disease by lowering your chances of developing blocked arteries. Resveratrol makes cells less likely to stick to the inner walls of your arteries.

While not yet attributed to a specific nutrient, eating nuts appears to lower your risk of developing gallstones. In fact, eating just one serving of nuts or peanut butter a week (that's right, I said per week, not day) significantly cut the risk of gallstones in study participants.

Diets high in unsaturated fats, specifically from peanuts, can lower your risk of heart disease considerably. Studies including moderate amounts of fat and peanuts in the diets have resulted in maintained levels of HDL or good cholesterol, lower triglyceride levels, and lower ratios of bad to good, or LDL to HDL, cholesterol. The improvements to cardiovascular health from these diets did not happen in the often-recommended low-fat diets.

Now I'm guessing you may be thinking, "Well, if I eat peanuts and peanut butter all the time, I'm going to blow up like an elephant." Not true, however. It turns out that a peanut-rich diet may in fact help you lose weight! Picture this: one group of folks followed a low-fat diet, about 20 percent of their total daily calories coming from fat, which isn't a heck of a lot, so their food choices were somewhat limited. Another group of people ate a moderate-fat diet, about 35 percent of calories coming from fat, with much of the fat coming from mono-unsaturated fat foods like peanuts, peanut butter, and nuts. Both groups ate about the same amount of calories. What do you think happened? Well, many of those folks in the low-fat group quit because they couldn't stick to the diet. Those who stuck it out lost about the same amount of weight as the moderate-fat, or nut, group, but weren't able to keep it off. In fact, after 2½ years, many of the nut people had kept most of their weight off, but many of the low-fat folks gained all their weight back and then some.

Kryptonite

Food allergies affect an estimated 1 percent of adults and 8 percent of children. Allergic reactions can range from a runny nose to a rash to a headache, up to the potentially fatal anaphylaxis, a rare allergic reaction that can cause difficulty breathing, a loss of consciousness, and sometimes even death. Peanuts and tree nuts (walnuts, pecans, etc.) are two of the nine most common food allergens. For this reason doctors recommend waiting to introduce these items into a child's diet until she is 18 to 24 months old. If there's a history of food allergies in your family, you may want to consider holding off on nuts until 2 or 3 years of age.

In addition, another study compared peanut eaters to nonpeanut eaters. While the men, women, and children who regularly ate peanuts or peanut butter ate more calories than nonpeanut eaters, they tended to have lower BMIs. So although they ate more, they were thinner. It's suspected that because the healthy fat-rich peanut foods are more satiating than low-fat, high-carb foods, it's much easier to stay with diets that include them. Taste also plays a role. Enjoying what you eat is important to enjoying life, but is crucial when trying to modify your eating habits and lose weight.

So go ahead and spread that peanut butter on your morning toast instead of butter. Or mix some peanuts with raisins for a high-protein, high-energy midafternoon pick-me-up. Or whip up a Thai-style peanut sauce for your chicken at dinner.

The Awe of Almonds

Are you ready to find out how almonds can be a joy in your diet?

Nutrition Information for 1 Ounce of Almonds (About 23 Nuts)

Calories	160
Total Fat	14 grams
Saturated Fat	1 gram
Trans Fat	0 grams

Cholesterol	0 milligrams
Sodium	0 milligrams
Total Carbohydrate	6 grams
Dietary Fiber	3 grams
Sugars	1 gram
Protein	6 grams
Calcium	8% Daily Value
Iron	6% Daily Value

Like the nuts before, almonds are full of a variety of nutrients. Some properties they share with walnuts and peanuts; other properties are unique to almonds.

Researchers recently looked at almonds to determine their antioxidant power. They found that almonds rank right up there with fruits and veggies for antioxidant power. In fact, almonds have as much of the flavonoids kaempferol and quercetin as broccoli and as much catechin as brewed tea. These are some of the most powerful of all flavonoids, offering protection from cell damage caused by oxidation. This enables them to help protect the body from both cardiovascular disease and age-related diseases.

Almonds are great sources of vitamin E. Vitamin E and the flavonoids work together to prevent LDL cholesterol oxidation, thereby decreasing the chances of cardiovascular disease.

Super Knowledge

Most of the flavonoids in almonds are found in their skin, while the vitamin E is in what's considered the meat of the nut. While both of these components provide benefits by themselves, their impact is greatened tremendously when eaten together. This isn't unusual. Often the health benefits of nutrients within foods are magnified by other nutrients within the food. This is one reason why eating whole foods is usually healthier than simply taking vitamin and mineral supplements.

Almonds contain large amounts of magnesium as well. One serving provides almost one quarter of your daily needs. Magnesium enables your blood vessels to work better, improving blood flow and maximizing the transport of oxygen and nutrients throughout your body. Also, having enough magnesium can help lessen the damage that a heart attack causes if you do have one.

As with peanuts, almonds help lower the chances of developing gallstones. So whether you choose to make almonds the only nut you eat or plan to include them in the variety of nuts you eat, they will give you protection from gallstones.

Like the other nuts, adding almonds to your diet won't necessarily put you in the fast lane to weight gain. A study comparing a low-fat, low-calorie, high-carbohydrate diet and a moderate-fat diet including almonds showed quite the opposite. While both diets included the same amount of calories and protein, they did not produce the same results. The almond-rich diet followers had much greater success than those on the low-fat diet. The almond eaters lost more weight, inches around their waist, and body fat. In fact, those eating almonds saw their blood pressure go down, too, but the nonalmond eaters' blood pressure stayed the same. Some of the dieters had diabetes and were able to cut down on their diabetic medicine. But only half of the low-fat dieters were able to do so, while almost all of the almond-eaters lowered their medication needs.

And I can't discuss almonds without mentioning their role in preventing heart disease. One study showed that a diet including a moderate amount of fat as well as foods like almonds, soy, oats, and beans lowered LDL cholesterol levels as much as 30 percent. That was the same reduction seen in people taking a popular type of cholesterol-lowering medicine known as statins. They should not, however, be considered a replacement for medication. And you should never change or stop any medication without speaking with your health-care professional first.

Plus, the only side effect was enjoying a delicious variety of foods on a regular basis.

If you're trying to lower your risk of heart disease and want to use almonds or other nuts to do so, you have two basic options. The first is that you can replace carbohydrates in your diet with nuts or nut butter. So instead of having foods like bread or crackers, try cutting the bread or crackers in half and put some peanut butter on them. This simple change will lower your chances of developing heart disease by about 30 percent. Your other option is just as easy. Replace saturated fats, those found mostly in animal products like meats and full-fat dairy foods, with an equal amount of nuts. For example, sprinkle a handful of nuts on a salad instead of cheese or meat. Doing so can cut your risk of heart disease by a whopping 45 percent!

The Least You Need to Know

- One serving of nuts a day is generally all that's needed to benefit nutritionally.

- A serving is usually one ounce, which is about a handful or one quarter cup.

- Many nuts contain as much disease-fighting antioxidant power as antioxidant-rich fruits and veggies.

- To lower your cholesterol, instead of simply cutting out fat, consider replacing unhealthy saturated fat-filled foods with healthy unsaturated fat-filled foods like nuts and nut butters.

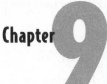

The Spices of Life

In This Chapter

- Need more fiber? Sprinkle some cinnamon on your food or drinks
- Reasons to turn up the heat in your food
- Peppermint leaves are more than a dessert garnish in fancy restaurants
- Some big things come out of very small packages

Spices add tantalizing aromas and fabulous flavors to the foods you eat, but did you ever think that they could improve your health? That's right, those tiny jars and tins in your kitchen cupboard are filled with all kinds of disease-fighting nutrients and phytochemicals. In fact, the contents of your spice rack may do more for your health than what's in your medicine cabinet.

Cinnamon

You may sprinkle it on top of your fancy coffee drink or mix it with your applesauce, but you might just want to think about using cinnamon a lot more.

Nutrition Information for 2 Teaspoons of Cinnamon

Calories	10
Total Fat	0 grams
Saturated Fat	0 grams
Trans Fat	0 grams
Cholesterol	0 milligrams
Sodium	0 milligrams
Total Carbohydrate	4 grams
Dietary Fiber	2 grams
Sugars	0 grams
Protein	0 grams
Vitamin C	2% Daily Value
Calcium	6% Daily Value
Iron	10% Daily Value

Cinnamon sticks are actually dried pieces of bark from the cinnamon tree. Grinding these sticks results in the powdery spice used in cooking and baking. The essential oils in this bark are where the health-producing substances are found.

Cinnamaldehyde is one of these substances. This component helps stop the unwanted clumping together of blood platelets. You need platelets to clump to stop the bleeding when you injure yourself. But clumps in your blood vessels lead to inadequate blood flow and increase the risk of having a heart attack or a stroke. By blocking this specific clumping, cinnamon can lower your risk of cardiovascular disease.

Surprisingly, cinnamon is also a good source of fiber and calcium. This provides another avenue for cinnamon to battle heart disease. Just 2 teaspoons contain as much fiber as a slice of whole-wheat bread and more than 50 milligrams of calcium. Both calcium and fiber bind with a substance called bile salts, which are produced by your liver. This bound mixture is then easily transported out of the body. Bile is made from cholesterol, and when it's removed from the body, the liver gets a message to make more bile. In order to do so, it must use more cholesterol, thus lowering the blood levels of cholesterol. The result is a decreased likelihood that you will develop heart disease.

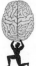

Super Knowledge

Cinnamon should be stored in a cool, dry, dark place. Ground cinnamon will stay fresh for about 6 months and cinnamon sticks will last about a year. An easy test for cinnamon's freshness is to smell it. If it doesn't have that sweet aroma anymore, it's time to buy new cinnamon.

Cinnamon is also involved in blood sugar control in people with diabetes. In diabetes, levels of the hormone insulin are inadequate, or the body's cells don't respond to it the way they should. This means that glucose, or the sugar in the blood, can't get into the cells where it's needed and instead continues to circulate in the blood, damaging some organs. Cinnamon helps your body's cells to use glucose more efficiently in two different ways. It does so by enhancing the work of the insulin receptors that let glucose get into the cells. On top of that, cinnamon hinders an enzyme that makes these receptors work incorrectly.

Another problem associated with diabetes is that it increases your risk of heart disease. Cinnamon plays a role in helping that as well. Studies have shown that in addition to lowering blood sugar levels, eating as little as one half teaspoon of cinnamon a day can also lower levels of total cholesterol, LDL cholesterol, and triglycerides.

One final interesting benefit of cinnamon is that it can help stop the growth of bacteria and fungi, including yeasts. This ability also helps to make cinnamon useful as a food preservative. In one study, just a few drops of cinnamon essential oil to carrot broth prevented the growth of a common food-poisoning bacteria for at least 60 days.

Not sure how to fit cinnamon into your diet? It's more versatile than you might think. In some cultures it's common to pair it with chocolate, so try sprinkling some in hot chocolate or mix a teaspoon or so into the next batch of brownies you make. For a more American flavor, mix some into oatmeal in the morning for a nutritious and delicious breakfast. When you want a little snack, mix cinnamon and honey and spread on toast. This will give you a double health bonus—keep reading to find out the benefits of honey in Chapter 10.

Some Like It Hot: Cayenne Pepper

If you already love your food to have a little kick, I'll give you more reasons to turn up the heat.

Nutrition Information for 2 Teaspoons of Cayenne Pepper

Calories	10
Total Fat	0.5 grams
Saturated Fat	0 grams
Trans Fat	0 grams
Cholesterol	0 milligrams
Sodium	0 milligrams
Total Carbohydrate	2 grams
Dietary Fiber	1 gram
Sugars	0 grams
Protein	0 grams
Vitamin A	30% Daily Value
Vitamin C	4% Daily Value
Iron	2% Daily Value

A substance called capsaicin is what gives cayenne pepper and all peppers their fire. And not surprisingly, the more capsaicin the pepper has, the hotter it is.

In addition to burning up your insides, capsaicin is responsible for several of cayenne pepper's health benefits. Have you ever noticed your nose running when you eat some good Mexican food, or any other spicy dish? That's capsaicin in action. It stimulates the mucus membranes in the nose and respiratory tract to help them drain. When you're healthy you may think it's an annoyance, but when you're suffering from a cold with a stuffed-up nose or congested lungs, it may just be your savior. In fact, capsaicin is similar to an ingredient in many cold medicines, but it works a lot faster at loosening things up and clearing out your stuffed-up nose or congested lungs. Think about that the next time you're under the weather.

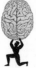

Super Knowledge

While eating capsaicin may be painful if you're not a fan of spicy food, it's actually a pain *reliever* in some circumstances. Creams containing capsaicin have been used to treat pain for people suffering from osteoarthritis and cluster headaches. Now, I'm not suggesting you start rubbing cayenne pepper all over your body, but you might want to check the ingredients the next time you're buying a pain cream and try one with capsaicin in it.

And while this isn't a direct action of capsaicin, it's certainly a beneficial result of eating peppers and foods containing them. Spicy food often brings with it a wave of heat flowing through your body. Well, believe it or not, in order for your body to turn up the temperature like that, it needs energy. Your body's energy source is calories. So when you eat hot peppers, your body actually burns more calories than usual. And it continues to burn calories at a higher rate for more than 20 minutes after you eat them. I'm not saying eating peppers is going to help you fit into your high school jeans overnight, but including cayenne pepper in your diet can be just one more step in helping you drop a few pounds.

Kryptonite

The heat from peppers is found primarily in the seeds and ribs that the seeds are on inside of the peppers. It can be pretty powerful. Whenever you work with peppers, be sure to wash your hands well before touching your eyes or any other mucus membrane. Better yet, wear rubber or latex gloves. Trust me, you don't want that pepper residue in your eyes.

Peppers are also a great source of vitamin A. Two teaspoons of cayenne pepper provide just under a third of your daily requirement. If you remember, vitamin A is needed for healthy tissue, like that lining the respiratory, digestive, and reproductive tracts as well as all other body cavities. Plus it's a powerful antioxidant and protects your body from free-radical damage that can lead to diseases like heart disease and certain cancers, just to name a couple.

Red chili peppers, including cayenne, have been shown to lower your risk of heart disease in other ways, too. They help to lower blood cholesterol and triglyceride levels. Cayenne and other red chili peppers also help the body dissolve a substance called *fibrin*, which is a key player in blood clot development.

def•i•ni•tion

> **Fibrin** is a protein that forms the basis of blood clots.

And here's one I bet will surprise you. If you or someone you've known has ever had a stomach ulcer, you may have thought that eating a lot of spicy foods was the cause. Well, I've got news for you. Hot chili peppers like cayenne may actually help prevent—that's right, I said prevent—stomach ulcers. They work in two ways. The first is by killing the bacteria you might have eaten that would cause an ulcer. The second is by kicking your stomach lining's cells into high gear. They cause these cells to release protective juices that help prevent ulcers from forming. So please don't give up cayenne pepper with the misguided idea that you'll lower your risk of developing a stomach ulcer. For that benefit, keep on eating the hot stuff.

You don't even need to be much of a cook to get more of this nutritious spice into your diet. Fill an empty pepper shaker with some and keep it on the table alongside your salt and pepper. That way it's right there to remind you to use it and convenient when you want to sprinkle some on your morning eggs, your soup at lunch, or your mashed potatoes or steamed veggies at dinner.

The Peppermint Twist

Fresh peppermint leaves are frequently used as a dessert garnish in restaurants, but there's so much more to them than just their pretty look.

Nutrition Information for 2 Tablespoons of Peppermint Leaves

Calories	2
Total Fat	0 grams
Saturated Fat	0 grams
Trans Fat	0 grams
Cholesterol	0 milligrams
Sodium	1 milligram
Total Carbohydrate	0 grams
Dietary Fiber	0 grams
Sugars	0 grams
Protein	0 grams

One of the most common uses for peppermint is improving stomach ailments. Peppermint relaxes smooth muscle, the type that surrounds the intestinal tract. When this muscle is relaxed, it's less likely to go into spasms and cause indigestion. Therefore peppermint and peppermint oil can be used to improve indigestion by itself, as well as indigestion as a symptom of irritable bowel syndrome (IBS). Other symptoms of IBS, such as muscle spasms, can be alleviated with peppermint as well.

Like cinnamon, peppermint oil can prevent the growth of a variety of bacteria. These include H. pylori, the bacteria that causes stomach ulcers, and bacteria referred to as MRSA that is resistant to some antibiotics, as well as the more commonly talked about salmonella and E. coli bacteria.

One component of peppermint is rosmarinic acid. This substance is an antioxidant and therefore protects cells from free-radical damage. However, it is also very beneficial in improving asthma. By slowing the production of chemicals that can cause inflammation and by increasing the production of substances that help to keep airways open, rosmarinic acid in peppermint helps make breathing much easier for asthma sufferers. In addition, peppermint has been shown to improve the stuffy and runny nose, sneezing, and nasal itching associated with allergic rhinitis—more commonly called hay fever.

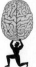

Super Knowledge

To store fresh peppermint, wrap the leaves in a damp paper towel and place inside a plastic bag. Store this little peppermint package in the refrigerator for several days. This is a great way to store any fresh herb.

Need some ideas for how to get more peppermint into your diet? If you have an upset stomach or a bit of indigestion, try drinking a cup of tea brewed with peppermint leaves. Or next time you make a fruit salad, which should be soon based on everything I told you in Chapter 2, chop up some fresh mint leaves to toss in with the fruit.

The Least You Need to Know

- Cinnamon, cayenne pepper, and peppermint do so much more than flavor your food.
- You don't need to eat large amounts of spices to obtain their numerous health benefits.
- Cayenne pepper doesn't cause stomach ulcers.
- Try some peppermint tea the next time your stomach isn't doing so well.

Chapter 10

How Sweet It Is

In This Chapter

- Sweet stuff can be good for you
- Honey for energy
- Yes, you can eat chocolate
- Why chocolate is the perfect candy to fill those little heart-shaped boxes

What a perfect ending for this book—the sweet stuff. Think of this chapter as the dessert after a meal made up of a plethora of information on other superfoods.

Oh, Honey, Honey

Who'd have guessed that the sticky substance that bees make from flower nectar they've eaten is not only something many of us eat, but is good for us, too?

Nutrition Information for 1 Tablespoon of Honey

Calories	60
Total Fat	0 grams
Saturated Fat	0 grams
Trans Fat	0 grams
Cholesterol	0 milligrams
Sodium	0 milligrams
Total Carbohydrate	17 grams
Dietary Fiber	0 grams
Sugars	16 grams
Protein	0 grams

I think the most interesting aspect of honey is its use as an aid in sports performance. It's long been known that carbohydrates maximize an athlete's ability while participating in sports, whether it be running, biking, football, tennis, or any other sport. Carbohydrates are the preferred food source because when compared to fats and protein, they are the group most efficiently converted to glucose by the body. Glucose is to your body what gas is to your car—it's the stuff that makes it go.

When you're exercising intensely, your body uses up the glucose circulating in your blood but also digs into glucose that is stored in your muscle for just such an occasion. Eating carbohydrates before exercising or participating in a sport ensures that the maximum amount of energy is available for your body to use. Eating them during an event helps to maintain a constant supply—this is especially important for an exercise or sport that lasts a long time. And eating carbs after you finish helps to replace all the energy your body used.

Honey is a great source of the needed energy. It's made up entirely of carbohydrates. Plus these carbs are in a form that is readily available and easily absorbed by your body. In addition, it has a slightly slower glycemic index than sugar, another readily available and easily absorbed energy source. This means that after you eat it, your blood sugar rises slowly and steadily. This is important for two reasons. During exercise, slow absorption allows for sustained energy versus a quick absorption that would give you a fast rise in blood sugar and energy but then lead to a sudden drop of both. After exercise, the slower absorption means better replacement of energy stores in the muscle. This means your muscles will have all the stored energy they need to enable you to exercise or participate in your sport at your maximum ability again the next day.

Honey also has antiseptic properties and can be beneficial in wound healing. Studies have shown that it helps in two ways. Honey can decrease the likelihood of infection in burns and open wounds. It can also speed healing. The reason honey helps isn't quite known, but there are a couple of ideas. Honey may absorb the water from the wound, which inhibits the growth of bacteria and fungi.

Also, honey contains an enzyme that creates an antiseptic when combined with water. Certainly, however, if you have a serious burn or injury, honey should not be used in place of seeking medical advice.

Kryptonite

While it is a superfood, honey should never be given to children under the age of 1. Honey may contain spores of the bacteria Clostridium botulinum. These spores can be found throughout the environment—the air, soil, dust, etc. And when it comes to honey, the spores can't be killed without destroying the honey. They cause no problems in healthy adults and children because the normal flora in your intestinal tract digests them. Infants, however, haven't yet developed this flora, and the bacteria can make them sick.

Symptoms of infant botulism include general muscle weakness, a weak cry, a feeble suck, and constipation. If you see these symptoms in an infant, contact a doctor.

Honey also contains antioxidants. These may play a role in wound healing because they inhibit the growth of common bacteria that cause infections in open wounds.

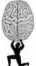

Honey can be spread on toast alone or mixed with cinnamon. It can also be used as a substitute for sugar in tea or in baking and cooking. It is sweeter than sugar, though, so you need to use only one half to three quarters of a cup of honey for every cup of sugar a recipe calls for. Also, because it's a liquid, cut the recipe's liquid down by one quarter of a cup. Lower the cooking temperature as well because honey browns foods quicker than sugar.

Yes, Chocolate Is a Superfood!

Yum, yum, yum! Like you needed a reason to eat chocolate.

Nutrition Information for 1.4 Ounces of Dark Chocolate (Semi-Sweet)

Calories	210
Total Fat	13 grams
Saturated Fat	8 grams

continues

Nutrition Information for 1.4 Ounces of Dark Chocolate (Semi-Sweet) (continued)

Cholesterol	5 milligrams
Sodium	0 milligrams
Total Carbohydrate	23 grams
Dietary Fiber	4 grams
Sugars	20 grams
Protein	2 grams
Iron	6% Daily Value

Nutrition Information for 1.4 Ounces of Milk Chocolate

Calories	210
Total Fat	12 grams
Saturated Fat	8 grams
Cholesterol	10 milligrams
Sodium	35 milligrams
Total Carbohydrate	23 grams
Dietary Fiber	1 gram
Sugars	20 grams
Protein	2 grams
Calcium	8% Daily Value
Iron	2% Daily Value

The big scuttlebutt about chocolate is how good it can be for your heart. Are they crazy? That creamy delight that's not too sweet, not too bitter, but just right? That perfect ending to any meal? That stuff's good for you? No way.

It's true! In fact, chocolate is so good for you that some folks rank it right up there with red wine for its benefits for your heart health.

Just like most of the other foods I've talked about, chocolate contains beneficial phytochemicals. Specifically, chocolate contains flavonoids including *epicatechin* and *catechin*. In fact, cocoa contains twice as much epicatechin as red wine and three times as much as tea.

The flavonoids in chocolate are quickly absorbed after you eat them. And they do all sorts of healthy things for you. As antioxidants they protect the body from damage by decreasing the oxidation of LDL cholesterol, lowering the chances of dangerous plaque forming and building up in your arteries.

def•i•ni•tion

Epicatechin is a flavonoid found primarily in cocoa, red wine, and green tea. It improves blood flow and is therefore beneficial for maintaining heart health.

Catechin is a flavonoid and powerful antioxidant. Its major source in the diet is white and green tea.

You may have heard of or been told yourself to take a baby aspirin to help your heart. Studies comparing aspirin to chocolate showed the same results in both. And just what were those results, you may ask? Both chocolate and aspirin decrease the activity of blood platelets. If you remember, these are the guys responsible for blood clotting. By decreasing their activity, chocolate allows for better blood flow and lowers your risk of developing blood clots, which in turn lowers your risk of having a heart attack or stroke.

Having healthy arteries is key to good cardiovascular health. Healthy arteries allow blood to flow easily when and where it's needed. Unhealthy arteries increase your vulnerability to heart attacks and strokes. The flavonoids in cocoa have been shown to improve the health of arteries, allowing for better blood flow and a lower risk of a cardiovascular emergency.

Generally, the more cocoa in a product, the more antioxidant power it has. Dark and baking chocolate tends to contain more flavonoids than milk chocolate, which has some of the cocoa replaced by milk or cream. Also, if you happen to be a baker, you may have heard the term Dutch or alkalinized cocoa. Cocoa that's been treated in that way also has less flavonoids and therefore less nutritional power than natural or nonalkalinized cocoa.

Different Types of Chocolate

Milk Chocolate	A mixture of chocolate liquor (a liquid form of chocolate made by grinding the center of shelled, fermented, dried, and roasted cocoa beans), cocoa butter, sugar, and milk or cream.
Dark Chocolate, also called Semi-sweet or Bitter-sweet	A mixture of chocolate liquor, cocoa butter, and sugar.
Unsweetened or Baking Chocolate	Pure chocolate liquor with no additions. Made by grinding cocoa beans until they are smooth.
White Chocolate	A mixture of cocoa butter, sugar, and milk or cream. Contains no chocolate liquor.
Cocoa	The powder obtained when the cocoa beans are ground after the cocoa butter has been removed. Since much of the fat is in the cocoa butter, cocoa powder contains very little fat.

Because milk chocolate contains cream or milk and sugar, much of the health benefits are outweighed by the extra fat and calories. To maximize your benefits, stick to the darker chocolates with the least additives.

Chocolate also contains fat, and not just any fat but that nasty saturated kind. But it turns out that the saturated fat found in chocolate is unique. One type of saturated fat in chocolate is called palmitic acid and it's your standard saturated fat that you don't want to eat too much of. Another type of saturated fat found in chocolate is stearic acid. This is the interesting one. While other saturated fats raise cholesterol, stearic acid doesn't. In fact, stearic acid has no effect on cholesterol at all. Chocolate also contains oleic acid, which is an unsaturated fat. It's the same kind found in olive oil and it actually helps lower cholesterol and LDL levels.

So of the three main fats in chocolate, one type is known to lower cholesterol and another has a neutral effect on blood cholesterol. And apparently the combination of the three sort of evens things out—studies have shown that diets including choc-olate and cocoa have no effect on blood cholesterol levels. If you're a chocolate lover like I am, that alone is cause to celebrate.

The Least You Need to Know

- Infants 12 months old or younger shouldn't be given honey.
- Consider some honey to give you energy before your next workout.
- Some chocolate now and then can easily fit into a healthy eating plan.
- Surprisingly, cocoa contains no fat and therefore isn't bad for your cholesterol.

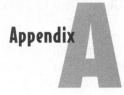

Glossary

alpha-carotene   A carotenoid and precursor to vitamin A.

amino acids   The building blocks of which proteins are made.

anaphylaxis   A severe and quickly occurring allergic reaction that can affect many parts of the body at once, including the skin, throat, and lungs. Symptoms include throat and tongue swelling, hives, and vomiting. It can cause difficulty breathing and a loss of consciousness, and could in rare instances cause death. Fortunately, it is rare and death occurs in only about 1 of every 2.5 million people per year.

antioxidants   Substances that protect your body's cells from the stress and damage done by free radicals. They may possibly reduce the risks of certain cancers and age-related diseases.

atherosclerosis   A thickening and hardening of artery walls due to fat deposits on their lining. It's responsible for a great deal of coronary artery/heart disease as well as strokes.

bacteria Microscopic living organisms that are practically everywhere: on the skin, in the intestines, air, soil, and more.

beta-carotene An antioxidant that is turned into vitamin A by the body. Among the several antioxidants that do this, beta-carotene is the easiest for the body to transform.

beta-cryptoxanthin Another of the carotenoids that the body converts to vitamin A.

carbohydrates The body's main source of energy. They include sugars, starches, and fiber.

carotenoids Strong antioxidants that may lower the risk of heart disease, some types of cancer, age-related eye diseases, and lung diseases. They are responsible for the vibrant orange and red colors of many vegetables.

cataract A cloudy layer that forms over the eye's lens. It causes blurry vision and light sensitivity.

catechin A flavonoid and powerful antioxidant. Its major source in the diet is white and green tea.

chocolate liquor A liquid form of chocolate made by grinding the center of shelled, fermented, dried, and roasted cocoa beans. Once cooled, it is often molded into blocks of unsweetened chocolate. Contains no alcohol.

collagen A protein that helps build connective tissue in your body.

DASH diet Dietary Approaches to Stop Hypertension. It's an eating plan high in fruits, veggies, and low-fat dairy foods that's low in fat, saturated fat, and cholesterol.

Diabetes Mellitus A chronic disease characterized by high levels of glucose, or sugar, in the blood. Consistent blood sugar elevation can damage the kidneys and eyes, to name a few of the complications of diabetes. There are three main types: Type 1, Type 2, and gestational. References to diabetes in this book are regarding Type 2. This type of diabetes is usually diagnosed later in life, although more and more young people are developing it. A major risk factor of this type of diabetes is being overweight or obese.

Dietary Reference Intake (DRI) A newer version of the RDA. Developed in 1995 to provide more information, the DRIs include the RDA; Adequate Intake (AI) for nutrients, for which no RDA has been set; Tolerable Upper Intake Levels (UL), which are to prevent excessive intakes of nutrients that can do harm when consumed in too large amounts; and the Estimated Average Requirements (EAR), which are expected to meet the needs of half the people in the age group.

edamame Fresh green soybeans. They are high in protein and fiber. Often found in the freezer section of most grocery stores.

ellagic acid A polyphenol that has antioxidant properties and helps reduce the risk of certain cancers.

endothelium   The inside lining of artery walls.

epicatechin   A flavonoid found primarily in cocoa, red wine, and green tea. It improves blood flow and is therefore beneficial for maintaining heart health.

fibrin   A protein that forms the basis of blood clots.

flash freezing   A super-quick way of freezing food to maintain flavor and nutrition.

flavonoids   The most powerful and abundant phytochemical group in your diet.

folate   A B-vitamin that plays a big role in preventing birth defects and producing red blood cells. It is also called folic acid.

free radicals   The by-product of the normal chemical reactions in the body. They damage cells and accelerate the development of age-related diseases and other diseases. Smoking, high exposure to pollution, and exposure to ultraviolet light (for example, sunbathing) increase free radical production.

fructose   A sugar found naturally in fruits.

gastritis   An inflammation of the stomach.

gastrointestinal tract   Also called the digestive tract. It's made up of all of the organs involved in digestion, including the mouth, stomach, and intestines.

glucose   The sugar that is the body's main source of energy.

Glycemic Index (GI)   A measure of how foods affect blood sugar levels and the body's insulin response after eating.

hesperetin   A flavonoid shown in animal studies to possess many health-promoting properties involving blood pressure, inflammation, and heart disease.

HDL   High-density lipoprotein. Referred to as "good" cholesterol, HDL helps rid cholesterol from the body.

homocysteine   An amino acid found in your blood. High levels of it coincide with a higher risk of heart disease.

indoles   Anti-cancer phytochemicals found in cruciferous vegetables.

inflammatory bowel syndrome (IBS)   An intestinal condition characterized by abdominal pain, bloating, and alternating constipation and diarrhea.

insoluble fiber   A part of plant-based foods that cannot be digested. It's found in wheat bran, whole grains, fruits, and vegetables, and it increases the rate of food going through the intestines.

insulin   The hormone responsible for regulating blood sugar by transporting the sugar from your blood to the various body tissues that need it for fuel.

iron   A mineral that is essential to obtain from your diet. It's used to make hemoglobin, which is the component in blood that carries oxygen throughout the body to where it's needed. Too much iron, however, can be dangerous, so don't go overboard with iron-rich foods or supplements.

isoflavones Compounds found in plants that faintly imitate the work of the reproductive hormone estrogen. They are also called phytoestrogens and are found in chickpeas and legumes, the soybean being the legume with the most.

isolated soy protein Created by removing most of the nonprotein components from soybeans, resulting in a product that is almost pure soy protein. It's used as an ingredient in foods such as energy bars to boost the nutritional quality.

isothiocyanates Anti-cancer phytochemicals found in cruciferous vegetables.

lactose The sugar in milk and milk products. It is broken down in the body by the enzyme lactase.

lactose intolerance A condition in which the body doesn't break down lactose due to low levels of lactase. This can result in stomach pain, bloating, gas, and/or diarrhea.

LDL Low-density lipoprotein. Often called "bad" cholesterol, it's responsible for the plaque buildup that narrows arteries and could lead to a heart attack or stroke.

lignans Plant compounds that work as both phytoestrogens and antioxidants. These attributes are responsible for many health benefits.

lutein   A carotenoid whose antioxidant powers work to benefit the eye and heart as well as help prevent cancer.

lycopene   An antioxidant in the carotenoid group of phytochemicals.

macula   Special eye tissue that helps tell your brain what your eye is seeing.

metabolic syndrome   A group of risk factors linked to heart disease and diabetes. The risk factors include high blood pressure, low HDL cholesterol, high blood sugar, high triglycerides, and abdominal fat.

mineral   An inorganic substance essential for the body to function properly.

miso   Fermented soybean paste mixed with a grain.

motor skills   The abilities needed to perform large movements such as walking and sitting as well as finer movements of the hands, wrists, fingers, and toes.

myricetin   A flavonoid shown to have anti-inflammatory and anti-cancer properties in studies. It's found in fruits and vegetables, primarily berries, grapes, parsley, and spinach.

naringenin   A flavonoid shown in animal studies to possess many health-promoting properties involving blood pressure, inflammation, and heart disease.

nutrients   Components in food that the body uses for energy, to build tissue, or to control body functions.

omega-3 fatty acids   A group of essential poly-unsaturated fats found primarily in fish oils, especially salmon, that lower blood cholesterol levels. The two main ones are EPA (eicosapentaenoic acid) and DHA (docosahexaenoic acid).

omega-6 fatty acids   A group of essential fatty acids that compete in the body with omega-3 fatty acids. They are found in cereals, whole-grain breads, most vegetable oils, and baked goods.

osteoporosis   A disease in which your bones become less dense and more porous. This some-times painful condition increases your chances of fracturing bones and makes your hips and spine especially vulnerable. Osteoporosis can affect men as well as women, and while it can start even when you're young, the results are usually seen when you reach your 60s or after.

oxidation   A chemical reaction in the body that produces free radicals and damages cells.

peptic ulcer   A hole in the lining of the digestive tract—esophagus, stomach, or intestines.

Percent Daily Value   The amount of the recom-mended needs of the nutrient that the named food in the described portion provides. It is based on the needs of a person eating 2,000 calories per day.

phytochemicals Compounds found in plants that aren't essential for the body to function but are beneficial in improving health or decreasing the risk of certain diseases.

phytoestrogens Plant substances that weakly replicate the action of the hormone estrogen.

plant sterols Plant-based substances that compete with cholesterol for absorption by the intestines. By doing so, they help lower cholesterol levels.

potassium A mineral involved in controlling blood pressure and regulating muscle contractions.

prebiotics Indigestible carbohydrates in foods that encourage the growth of good bacteria in the intestines.

probiotics Living microorganisms that benefit your health beyond the basic strong body building when they are eaten in certain amounts.

proteins Substances that build and maintain structures in the body such as bone and skin, and regulate processes like fighting infection. The body can also use them for energy. Mostly found in meats and dairy products, they are also in grains, vegetables, and legumes.

quercetin The major flavonoid in the diet. Those who eat the most foods containing it have a decreased risk of asthma and lung cancer, and lower death from heart disease.

Recommended Daily Allowance (RDA) The amount of an essential nutrient, such as a vitamin or mineral, needed by most healthy people for adequate growth. They are established by the National Academy of Sciences and were first developed in 1941. Also called the recommended dietary allowance.

resveratrol An antioxidant found in high amounts in red wine, grapes, raspberries, and peanuts.

saturated fat A fat that is solid at room temperature, like butter and meat fat. It raises cholesterol levels.

serotonin A neurotransmitter involved in the regulation of appetite, sleep, and mood.

soluble fiber A part of plant-based foods that cannot be digested. It's found in oats, beans, fruits, and vegetables and it slows the rate of food going through the intestines.

sulforaphane An isothiocyanate found in broccoli and broccoli sprouts.

tempeh Cooked, whole soybeans mixed with a grain and cultured with an edible mold.

tofu Cooked soybeans puréed into a curd.

trans fat A type of fatty acid created when liquid fats, or oils, are solidified through a process called partial hydrogenation. This is done to make the fat more stable and increase its shelf life. Trans fats are far worse than the dreaded saturated fat because trans fats raise the LDL or bad cholesterol. Trans fats are found in shortening, solid or stick margarines, crackers, baked goods, and other snack foods.

triglycerides   The major form of fat in food as well as in the body. Its blood levels are often measured at the same time that your cholesterol levels are.

tryptophan   One of the 10 essential amino acids the body uses for protein synthesis.

ulcerative colitis   An inflammation of the colon.

unsaturated fat   A fat that is liquid at room temperature, like olive or canola oil. There are two types, polyunsaturated and monounsaturated. They tend to lower cholesterol levels.

vitamin   An organic substance that the body needs in very small amounts to function properly. Vitamins can come from plant or animal foods. In addition, the body has the ability to manufacture some vitamins, such as vitamins D and K.

zeaxanthin   A carotenoid that works as an antioxidant, protecting the eyes and preventing certain cancers. It's found in green, leafy vegetables and yellow and orange fruits and vegetables.

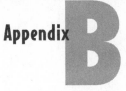

Dietary Reference Intakes for Selected Vitamins and Minerals

The following dietary reference intake recommendations were developed by the Food and Nutrition Board of the Institute of Medicine. Note that they apply to adults age 19 and above.

Age	Vitamin A (ug/d)	Vitamin C (mg/d)	Vitamin D (mg/d)	Vitamin E (ug/d)	Vitamin K (mg/d)
Males					
19 to 30	900	90	5	15	120
31 to 50	900	90	5	15	120
51 to 70	900	90	10	15	120
71 and above	900	90	15	15	120
Females					
19 to 30	700	75	5	15	90
31 to 50	700	75	5	15	90
51 to 70	700	75	10	15	90
71 and above	700	75	15	15	90

Age	Vitamin A (ug/d)	Vitamin C (mg/d)	Vitamin D (mg/d)	Vitamin E (ug/d)	Vitamin K (mg/d)
		Pregnant			
19 to 30	770	85	5	15	90
31 to 50	770	85	5	15	90
		Lactating			
19 to 30	1,300	120	5	19	90
31 to 50	1,300	120	5	19	90

ug/d= micrograms per day, mg/d= milligrams per day

Age	Thiamin (mg/d)	Riboflavin (mg/d)	Niacin (mg/d)	Vitamin B6 (mg/d)	Folate (ug/d)
Males					
19 to 30	1.2	1.3	16	1.3	400
31 to 50	1.2	1.3	16	1.3	400
51 to 70	1.2	1.3	16	1.7	400
71 and above	1.2	1.3	16	1.7	400
Females					
19 to 30	1.1	1.1	14	1.3	400
31 to 50	1.1	1.1	14	1.3	400
51 to 70	1.1	1.1	14	1.5	400
71 and above	1.1	1.1	14	1.5	400

Age	Thiamin (mg/d)	Riboflavin (mg/d)	Niacin (mg/d)	Vitamin B6 (mg/d)	Folate (ug/d)
Pregnant					
19 to 30	1.4	1.4	18	1.9	600
31 to 50	1.4	1.4	18	1.9	600
Lactating					
19 to 30	1.4	1.6	17	2.0	500
31 to 50	1.4	1.6	17	2.0	500

ug/d= micrograms per day, mg/d= milligrams per day

Age	Vitamin B12 (ug/d)	Calcium (mg/d)	Iron (mg/d)	Magnesium (mg/d)	Zinc (mg/d)
		Males			
19 to 30	2.4	1,000	8	400	11
31 to 50	2.4	1,000	8	420	11
51 to 70	2.4	1,200	8	420	11
71 and above	2.4	1,200	8	420	11
		Females			
19 to 30	2.4	1,000	18	310	8
31 to 50	2.4	1,000	18	320	8
51 to 70	2.4	1,200	8	320	8
71 and above	2.4	1,200	8	320	8

Age	Vitamin B12 (ug/d)	Calcium (mg/d)	Iron (mg/d)	Magnesium (mg/d)	Zinc (mg/d)
		Pregnant			
19 to 30	2.6	1,000	27	350	11
31 to 50	2.6	1,000	27	360	11
		Lactating			
19 to 30	2.8	1,000	9	310	12
31 to 50	2.8	1,000	9	320	12

ug/d= micrograms per day, mg/d= milligrams per day

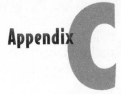

Internet Resources

About Seafood
www.aboutseafood.com

Almond Board of California
www.almondsarein.com

American Dietetic Association
www.eatright.org
1-800-877-1600

Beans for Health
www.beansforhealth.com

California Strawberry Commission
www.calstrawberry.com

California Walnuts
www.walnuts.org

Center for Science in the Public Interest
www.cspinet.org

Cherry Marketing Institute
www.cherrymkt.org

Cooking Light
www.cookinglight.com

Cranberry Institute
www.cranberryinstitute.com

Eating Well
www.eatingwell.com

Flax Council of Canada
www.flaxcouncil.ca

Flax RD
www.flaxrd.com

Healthier US
www.heatlhierus.gov

International Food Information Council
www.ific.org
202-296-6540

Light & Tasty
www.lightandtasty.com

Lipton Tea
www.lipton.com

McCormick
www.mccormick.com

Meal Makeover Moms
www.mealmakeovermoms.com

My Pyramid
www.mypyramid.gov

National Dairy Council
www.nationaldairycouncil.org

National Honey Board
www.honey.com

National Turkey Federation
www.eatturkey.com

Nutrition.gov
www.nutrition.gov

Peanut Institute
www.peanut-institute.org

Produce for Better Health Foundation
www.5aday.org

Quaker Oatmeal
www.quakeroatmeal.com

Salada
www.greentea.com

Six O'clock Scramble
www.thescramble.com

Supermarket Savvy
www.supermarketsavvy.com

United Soybean Board
www.soybean.org

United States Department of Agriculture
www.usda.gov

United States Department of Health and Human Services
www.hhs.gov

United States Food and Drug Administration/ Center for Food Safety and Applied Nutrition
www.cfsan.fda.gov

Vegetarian Resource Group
www.vrg.org

Welch's
www.welchs.com

Wild Blueberries
www.wildblueberries.com

World's Healthiest Foods
www.whfoods.org

Recommended Books

American Dietetic Association and Roberta Larson Duyuff. *American Dietetic Association Complete Food and Nutrition Guide.* Hoboken: Wiley, 2002.

Bixxex, Janice, Liz Weiss, and Laura Coyle. *The Mom's Guide to Meal Makeovers: Improving the Way Your Family Eats, One Meal at a Time.* New York: Broadway, 2003.

Cain, Anne C., and Anne C. Chappell. *Cooking Light Superfast Suppers: Speedy Solutions for Dinner Dilemmas.* Birmingham: Oxmoor House, 2003.

Clark, Nancy. *Nancy Clark's Sports Nutrition Guidebook, 3rd Edition.* Champaign: Human Kinetics Publishers, 2003.

Dunford, Marie. *Nutrition Logic: Food First, Supplements Second.* Kingsburg: Pink Robin Publishing, 2003.

Heroux, Cindy. *The Manual That Should Have Come with Your Body.* Oviedo: Speaking of Wellness, 2003.

Melina, Vesanto, Dina Aronson, and Jo Stepaniak. *Food Allergy Survival Guide: Surviving and Thriving with Food Allergies and Sensitivities.* Summertown: Healthy Living Publications, 2004.

Office of Disease Prevention and Health Promotion. *A Healthier You: Based on the Dietary Guidelines for Americans.* Office of Disease Prevention and Health, 2005.

Otten, Jennifer J., Jennifer Pitzi Hellwig, and Linda D. Meyers. *Dietary Reference Intakes: The Essential Guide to Nutrient Requirements.* National Academies Press, 2006.

Reseck, Heather Houck. *Fix-It-Fast: Vegetarian Cookbook.* Hagerstown: Review & Herald Publishing, 2002.

Romanoff, Jim. *The Eating Well Healthy in a Hurry Cookbook: 150 Delicious Recipes for Simple, Everyday Suppers in 45 Minutes or Less.* Woodstock: Countryman, 2006.

Sass, Cynthia, and Denise Maher. *Your Diet is Driving Me Crazy: When Food Conflicts Get in the Way of Your Love Life.* New York: Marlowe & Company, 2004.

Ward, Elizabeth M. *The Complete Idiot's Guide to Feeding Your Baby and Toddler.* Indianapolis: Alpha Books, 2005.

———. *The Pocket Idiot's Guide to the New Food Pyramids.* Indianapolis: Alpha Books, 2006.

Weinhofen, Donna L. *Mom's Updated Quick Meals Recipe Box: 250 Family Favorites in Thirty Minutes or Less.* Avon: Adams Media Corporation, 2006.

Zied, Elisa, and Ruth Winter. *So What Can I Eat?!: How to Make Sense of the New Dietary Guidelines for Americans and Make Them Your Own.* Hoboken: Wiley, 2006.

Index

A

ALA (essential fatty acid), 108, 131-133, 135
almonds
    health benefits, 149-152
    nutritional information, 148-149
anthocyanidins, 15-16
antioxidants
    berries, 12
    beta-carotene, 36
    carotenoids, 32
    cherries, 26
    defining characteristics, 12
    ellagic acid, 18, 22
    lycopene, 38
    resveratrol, 71
    saponin, 72
    strawberries, 21
arthritis, benefits of cherries, 27-28
atherosclerosis, 65

B

"bad" versus "good" foods, 1-4

beans
    health benefits, 113-116
    My Pyramid recommendations, 5
    nutritional information, 112
    plant sterols, 115
    prebiotics, 114
berries, 11
    antioxidants, 12
    blueberries
        health benefits, 17
        nutritional information, 14
        Oxygen Radical Absorbance Capacity, 15
    cranberries, 22-25
        health benefits, 23-25
        nutritional information, 23
    fresh versus frozen, 12-13
    phytochemicals, 12
    strawberries
        antioxidants, 21
        fiber content, 20-21
        folate, 19
        health benefits, 19-22

nutritional information, 17-18
potassium content, 21
beta-carotene, 36
beta-cryptoxanthin sources, 49-50
beta-glucan, 125
beverages. *See* drinks
blood pressure, high blood pressure, 127
blue/purple fruits, 61
blue/purple vegetables, 61
blueberries
health benefits, 15-17
nutritional information, 14
Oxygen Radical Absorbance Capacity, 15
body mass index (BMI) measurements, 128-129
broccoli
health benefits, 43
nutritional information, 41-43
sulforaphane content, 43

C

C-reactive proteins, 135
calcium sources
spinach, 48
yogurt, 98
canned fruits, 12
capsaicin, 158
carbohydrates, 98
carotenoids, 32
carrots
health benefits, 56
nutritional information, 55
catechin, 171
cayenne pepper
health benefits, 158-161
nutritional information, 157-158
cherries
health benefits, 27-29
nutritional information, 26-27
chocolate
flavonoids, 171
health benefits, 169-174
nutritional information, 169-170
types, 173
cinnamon
health benefits, 154-157
nutritional information, 154
storage, 155
cooking tips
tofu, 92
vegetables, 44
cranberries, 22-25
health benefits, 23-25
nutritional information, 23

D

DHA, 111
diabetes, 7-8, 28
diverticulitis, 135
drinks
  grape juice, 63-70
    purple Concord
      grape juice, 64-67
    white Niagara
      grape juice, 67-70
  red wine
    health benefits,
      70-74
    nutritional infor-
      mation, 70
  tea, 74-79
    health benefits,
      76-79
    nutritional infor-
      mation, 75-76

E-F

edamame, nutritional
  information, 87-88
eicosanoids, 107
ellagic acid, 18, 22
epicatechin, 171

fats
  ALA (essential fatty
    acid), 108, 131-133,
    135
  omega-3 fatty acids,
    107-108

defining character-
  istics, 108
flax, 130-135
health benefits,
  108-111
omega-6 fatty acids,
  107-108
saturated fats, 134
trans fats, 134
fiber
  beta-glucans, 125,
    128-129
  oats, 125, 128-129
  strawberries, 20-21
fibrin, 160
fish, salmon
  health benefits,
    108-111
  nutritional informa-
    tion, 106
  omega-3 fatty acids,
    107-108, 111
  omega-6 fatty acids,
    108
flavonoids, 15-16
  catechin, 171
  cranberries, 23
  epicatechin, 171
  hesperetin, 59
  myricetin, 16
  naringenin, 59
  quercetin, 18, 21
flavonols
  anthocyanidins, 15-16
  health benefits, 15-17
  myricetin, 16

proanthocyanidins,
15-16
flax
    health benefits,
    131-136
    lignans, 131-132
    nutritional informa-
    tion, 130-131
    omega-3 fatty acids,
    130-135
flour (soy flour), nutri-
tional information,
95-96
folate, 19, 145
free radicals, 28
fresh versus frozen fruits,
12
frozen versus fresh fruits,
12
fructose, 69
fruits
    blue/purple fruits, 61
    blueberries
        health benefits,
        15-17
        nutritional infor-
        mation, 14
    canned, 12
    cherries
        health benefits,
        27-29
        nutritional infor-
        mation, 26-27
    cranberries, 22-25
        health benefits,
        23-25

nutritional infor-
    mation, 23
fresh versus frozen, 12
green fruits, 61
My Pyramid recom-
    mendations, 5
orange fruits, 60-61
red fruits, 60
strawberries
    antioxidants, 21
    fiber content, 20-21
    folate, 19
    health benefits,
    19, 22
    nutritional infor-
    mation, 17-18
    potassium content,
    21
white fruits, 61-62
yellow fruits, 60-61

G

gastrointestinal tract, 100
glucose, 69
"good" versus "bad"
    foods, 1-4
gout, 27
grains
    flax
        health benefits,
        131-136
        lignans, 131-132
        nutritional infor-
        mation, 130-131

omega-3 fatty acids,
130-135
My Pyramid recom-
mendations, 5
oats, 123-129
health benefits,
124-129
nutritional infor-
mation, 124
grape juice, 63-70
purple Concord grape
juice, 64
health benefits,
65-67
nutritional infor-
mation, 64-65
white Niagara grape
juice, 67
health benefits,
68-70
nutritional infor-
mation, 67-68
green fruits, 61
green vegetables, 61
broccoli
health benefits, 43
nutritional infor-
mation, 41-43
sulforaphane con-
tent, 43
lutein, 39-40
spinach
health benefits,
46-48
nutritional infor-
mation, 44-46
vitamin K content, 40

H

HDL (high-density-
lipoprotein), 24
health benefits
almonds, 149-152
beans, 113-116
blueberries, 15-17
broccoli, 43
carrots, 56
cayenne pepper,
158-161
chocolate, 169-174
cherries, 27-29
cinnamon, 154-157
cranberries, 23-25
flavonoids, 15-16
flavonols, 15-17
flax, 131-136
honey, 166-169
oats, 124-129
omega-3 fatty acids,
108-111
oranges, 57-59
peanuts, 144-148
peppermint, 162-163
pumpkin, 54
purple Concord grape
juice, 65-67
red peppers, 35-38
red wine, 70-74
soy, 83-86
spinach, 46-48
strawberries, 19-22
sweet potatoes, 51-52
tea, 76-79
tomatoes, 38-39

turkey, 118-121
walnuts, 138-142
white Niagara grape
    juice, 68-70
yogurt, 98-103
healthy eating plans
    My Pyramid recom-
        mendations, 4-6
        fruits, 5
        grains, 5
        meats and beans, 5
        milk products, 5
        vegetables, 5
    Percent Daily Values,
        6-7
hesperetin, 59
high-density-lipoprotein.
    See HDL
high blood pressure, 127
homocysteine, 20, 145
honey
    health benefits,
        166-169
    nutritional informa-
        tion, 166
    precautions, 168

I

indoles, 42
inflammatory bowel syn-
    drome, 102
insomnia, 27
iron sources, spinach, 48
irritable bowel syndrome,
    162

isoflavones, soy, 82-83
isothiocyanates, 42

J-K

juices, grape juice, 63-70
    purple Concord grape
        juice, 64-67
    white Niagara grape
        juice, 67-70

L

l-arginine, 140
lactose intolerance, 90
LDL (low-density-
    lipoprotein), 24
lignans, 131-132
low-density-lipoprotein.
    See LDL
lutein, green vegetables,
    39-40
lycopene, 38

M

meats, My Pyramid rec-
    ommendations, 5
melatonin, 138
milk products
    My Pyramid recom-
        mendations, 5
    soymilk
        lactose intolerance
            and, 90

nutritional infor-
mation, 89-90
yogurt, 96-103
calcium content, 98
health benefits,
98-103
nutritional infor-
mation, 97
probiotics, 99-101
protein content, 97
miso, 92
My Pyramid recommen-
dations
fruits, 5
grains, 5
healthy eating plans,
4-6
meats and beans, 5
milk products, 5
vegetables, 5
myricetin, 16, 47

N

naringenin, 59
niacin sources, 118
nutritional information
almonds, 148-149
beans, 112
blueberries, 14
broccoli, 41-43
carrots, 55
cayenne pepper,
157-158
cherries, 26-27
chocolate, 169-170

cinnamon, 154
cranberries, 23
flax, 130-131
honey, 166
oats, 124
oranges, 57
peanuts, 142-144
peppermint, 161
pumpkin, 52-53
purple Concord grape
juice, 64-65
red peppers, 34-35
red wine, 70
salmon, 106
soy products, 86-96
edamame, 87-88
miso, 92
soy flour, 95-96
soy nuts, 94-95
soymilk, 89-90
tempeh, 93-94
tofu, 91
spinach, 44-46
strawberries, 17-18
sweet potatoes, 50-51
tea, 75-76
tomatoes, 37
turkey, 117-118
walnuts, 138
white Niagara grape
juice, 67-68
yogurt, 97
nuts
almonds
health benefits,
149-152

nutritional infor-
mation, 148-149
peanuts
health benefits,
144-148
nutritional infor-
mation, 142-144
soy nuts, 94-95
walnuts, 137
health benefits,
138-142
nutritional infor-
mation, 138

O

oats, 123-129
fiber content, 125-129
health benefits,
124-129
nutritional informa-
tion, 124
omega-3 fatty acids, 107
defining characteris-
tics, 108
flax, 130-135
health benefits,
108-111
omega-6 fatty acids,
107-108
orange fruits, 60-61
orange vegetables, 49-57,
60-61
beta-cryptoxanthin
content, 49-50

carrots
health benefits, 56
nutritional infor-
mation, 55
pumpkin, 55
health benefits, 54
nutritional infor-
mation, 52-53
sweet potatoes
health benefits,
51-52
nutritional infor-
mation, 50-51
oranges
health benefits, 57-59
nutritional informa-
tion, 57
vitamin C content,
57-59
oxidation, 24
oxidative stress, 12
Oxygen Radical Absor-
bance Capacity, 15

P–Q

palmitic acid, 174
peanuts
health benefits,
144-148
nutritional informa-
tion, 142-144
pepper (cayenne pepper)
health benefits,
158-161

nutritional information, 157-158
peppermint
health benefits, 162-163
nutritional information, 161
storage, 163
peppers (red), 33-38
health benefits, 35-38
nutritional information, 34-35
Percent Daily Values, 6-7
phytochemicals
berries, 12
beta-cryptoxanthin, 50
cherries, 26
flavonoids, 15-16
indoles, 42
isothiocyanates, 42
plant sterols, 115
potassium sources, 21
prebiotics, 114
precautions with honey, 168
proanthocyanidins, 15-16
probiotics, 99-101
protein sources
beans, 112-116
health benefits, 113-116
nutritional information, 112
plant sterols, 115
prebiotics, 114
C-reactive protein, 135

salmon
health benefits, 108-111
nutritional information, 106
omega-3 fatty acids, 107-108, 111
omega-6 fatty acids, 108
turkey
health benefits, 118-121
nutritional information, 117-118
tryptophan, 119-120
yogurt, 97
pumpkin, 52-55
health benefits, 54
nutritional information, 52-53
purple Concord grape juice
health benefits, 65-67
nutritional information, 64-65

quercetin, 18

R

RDA (Recommended Daily Allowance), 35
Recommended Daily Allowance. *See* RDA
red fruits, 60

red vegetables, 33, 60
  peppers, 33-38
    health benefits,
      35-38
    nutritional infor-
      mation, 34-35
  tomatoes
    health benefits,
      38-39
    lycopene, 38
    nutritional infor-
      mation, 37
red wine
  health benefits, 70-74
  nutritional informa-
    tion, 70
resveratrol, 71, 146

S

salmon
  health benefits,
    108-111
  nutritional informa-
    tion, 106
  omega-3 fatty acids,
    107-108, 111
  omega-6 fatty acids,
    108
saponin, 72
saturated fats, 134
serotonin, 119
soy
  eating plans and, 96
  edamame, 87-88

health benefits, 83-86
isoflavones, 82-83
miso, 92
nutritional informa-
  tion, 86-87
soy flour, 95-96
soy nuts, 94-95
soymilk
  lactose intolerance
    and, 90
  nutritional infor-
    mation, 89-90
tempeh, 93-94
tofu, 90-92
  cooking tips, 92
  nutritional infor-
    mation, 91
soymilk
  lactose intolerance
    and, 90
  nutritional informa-
    tion, 89-90
spices
  cayenne pepper
    health benefits,
      158-161
    nutritional infor-
      mation, 157-158
  cinnamon
    health benefits,
      154-157
    nutritional infor-
      mation, 154
  peppermint
    health benefits,
      162-163

nutritional information, 161
  storage, 163
spinach
  calcium content, 48
  health benefits, 46-48
  iron content, 48
  nutritional information, 44-46
stearic acid, 174
storage
  cinnamon, 155
  peppermint, 163
strawberries
  antioxidants, 21
  fiber content, 20-21
  folate, 19
  health benefits, 19-22
  nutritional information, 17-18
  potassium content, 21
sulforaphane sources, 43
sweet potatoes
  health benefits, 51-52
  nutritional information, 50-51
sweets
  chocolate
    flavonoids, 171
    health benefits, 169-174
    nutritional information, 169-170
    types, 173
honey
  health benefits, 166-169
  nutritional information, 166
  precautions, 168

T

tea, 74-79
  health benefits, 76-79
  nutritional information, 75-76
tempeh, 93-94
tofu, 90-92
  cooking tips, 92
  nutritional information, 91
tomatoes
  health benefits, 38-39
  lycopene, 38
  nutritional information, 37
trans fats, 134
tryptophan, 119-120
turkey
  health benefits, 118-121
  nutritional information, 117-118
  tryptophan, 119-120

U–V

ulcerative colitis, 102
urinary tract infections, 24

variety, importance of, 7-9
vegetables, 31-33
    blue/purple vegetables, 61
    cooking tips, 44
    green vegetables, 61
        broccoli, 41-43
        lutein, 39-40
        spinach, 44-48
        vitamin K content, 40
    My Pyramid recommendations, 5
    orange vegetables, 49-57, 60-61
        beta-cryptoxanthin content, 49-50
        carrots, 55-56
        pumpkin, 52-55
        sweet potatoes, 50-52
    red vegetables, 60
        peppers, 33-38
        tomatoes, 37-39
    white vegetables, 61-62
    yellow vegetables, 60-61
vitamin C sources, 57-59
vitamin K sources, 40

W–X

walnuts, 137
    health benefits, 138-142
    nutritional information, 138
white fruits, 61-62
white Niagara grape juice
    health benefits, 68-70
    nutritional information, 67-68
white vegetables, 61-62
wine
    red wine, 70
        health benefits, 70-74
        nutritional information, 70

Y–Z

yellow fruits, 60-61
yellow vegetables, 60-61
yogurt, 96-103
    calcium content, 98
    health benefits, 98-103
    nutritional information, 97
    probiotics, 99-101
    protein content, 97

zeaxanthin, 49
zinc sources, 120